Praise for

ROUGH MAGIC

"Miranda Newman's memoir about living with borderline personality disorder does two critical things by combining raw and witty
narrative with fact-based analysis: it shares a personal account of
navigating the unnecessarily complex mental health care system
in Canada and sheds light on the often stigmatized disorder. It's
books like this one that help make much-needed social and public
policy changes."
—**Sheima Benembarek, author of** *Halal Sex*

"*Rough Magic* is an important work gently but firmly asking the
reader to put themselves in the shoes of people with BPD and come
for a walk. Newman is a capable and experienced guide through
this terrain, deftly interweaving poetic recountings of a lifetime of
her own experiences with a rigorous and detailed analysis of BPD,
from its troubled beginning as a form of non-diagnosis to its dis-
appointing present as a highly stigmatized illness doctors are afraid
to even diagnose, while making room for a future full of growth and
healing at the personal, institutional, and societal levels."
—**Alex Manley, author of** *The New Masculinity*

"There are so few memoirs like *Rough Magic*: intimate, perspicacious, heartbreaking, and, ultimately, hopeful. Miranda Newman is an exceptional, fearless storyteller. We've been waiting for a writer like her, and finally, here she is."
—**Scaachi Koul, author of *One Day We'll All Be Dead and None of This Will Matter***

"Equal parts heartbreaking and hopeful, Miranda Newman's revelatory *Rough Magic* gives readers generous insight into an oft-misunderstood diagnosis. Blending personal history and broader cultural insight, Newman breaks down stigma, combats myths, and deftly reveals both the struggles and unexpected joys of living with BPD. Brimming with life, this brave, beautiful, and deeply moving book will stay with you long after you're done. *Rough Magic* is a genuine triumph."
—**Stacey May Fowles, author of *The Invitation***

"*Rough Magic* is at once an honest, heartfelt memoir and a piece of incisive nonfiction—both facets combine to present a riveting account of an often misunderstood disorder penned with bracing sincerity by Miranda Newman, who has lived-in experience."
—**Craig Davidson, author of *Cascade***

ROUGH MAGIC

ROUGH MAGIC

Living with Borderline Personality Disorder

MIRANDA NEWMAN

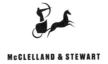

McCLELLAND & STEWART

Library and Archives Canada Cataloguing in Publication

Title: Rough magic : living with borderline personality disorder /
Miranda Newman.
Names: Newman, Miranda, author.
Identifiers: Canadiana (print) 20230485448 | Canadiana (ebook) 20230485464 |
ISBN 9780771006760 (softcover) | ISBN 9780771006838 (EPUB)
Subjects: LCSH: Newman, Miranda. | LCSH: Newman, Miranda—Mental
health. | LCSH: Borderline personality disorder—Patients—Canada—
Biography. | LCSH: Borderline personality disorder—Canada—Popular works. |
LCGFT: Autobiographies.
Classification: LCC RC569.5.B67 N49 2024 | DDC 616.85/8520092—dc23

Cover design by Jennifer Griffiths
Cover art: Miquel Llonch/Stocksy
Typeset in Heldane by Terra Page
Printed in Canada

McClelland & Stewart,
a division of Penguin Random House Canada Limited,
a Penguin Random House Company
www.penguinrandomhouse.ca

1 2 3 4 5   28 27 26 25 24

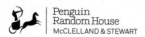

Penguin
Random House
McCLELLAND & STEWART

For my grandparents.

"This rough magic
I here abjure, and when I have required
Some heavenly music, which even now I do,
To work mine end upon their senses that
This airy charm is for, I'll break my staff,
Bury it certain fathoms in the earth,
And deeper than did ever plummet sound
I'll drown my book."

—WILLIAM SHAKESPEARE, *The Tempest*

". . . it was as if they didn't have emotional skin. As
if they had suffered from third-degree burns all over
their body. Even the lightest touch was excruciat-
ingly painful, and they lived in environments where
everyone kept poking at them."

—MARSHA LINEHAN, *Building a Life Worth Living*

CONTENTS

PSYCHIC BLEEDING

The sandy-haired admitting psychiatrist, Rick—which isn't his real name but a pseudonym, which I use for many other people who appear in this book—smiled gently at me over his half-moon-shaped glasses. I had just finished cataloguing my personal and medical history in the recycled air of a hospital meeting room, a routine so familiar from twelve years of seeking mental health care that reciting my symptoms felt like muscle memory. My partner, M., waited beyond the door in a locked lounge at Toronto's largest mental health hospital, the Centre for Addiction and Mental Health (CAMH). The waiting room, papered with AWOL risk signs, was named after a notable philanthropist I used to see at the boozy candlelit literary galas I coordinated during a more functional time in my life.

"I feel like it's worth mentioning that you're a lot more self-aware than most of the patients I see," Rick said. His hands rested on top of a manila folder, the only clutter in an otherwise sterile and featureless room. He wore a collared shirt, eschewing the lab coat uniform sported by so many of his colleagues. "You definitely have symptoms of PTSD. I was wondering, though, has anyone ever suggested that you might have borderline personality disorder?"

By twenty-seven years old, it had taken three hospitalizations; countless hours in waiting rooms that smelled of disinfectant mingled with piss; several legal forms that allowed medical professionals to detain me against my will for psychiatric assessment; so many drug counsellors, nurses, occupational therapists, and psychologists that their faces fused together in my mind; gallons of my tears; moderate liver damage; and a pint or so of blood to find a diagnosis that might fit my symptoms. In the days leading up to my hospitalization, these symptoms included a swarm of suicidal urges so powerful I had to hit the sides of my head with my fists to try to stop the chaos. I felt aimless in my work, unsure of what my goals were or where my life choices were leading me. I didn't know who I was or why I was living. I began to believe my partner, despite all evidence to the contrary, wanted me dead and was trying to push me to suicide through unspoken tests and intentional thoughtlessness. This activated my fear of abandonment, which sent panic attack after panic attack crashing over me in steady waves. I relied on weed too frequently to dull the sharp edges of my thoughts. I was plagued by fleeting mood swings so intense they caused physical discomfort. I slipped outside my body into a grey place away from any feeling until it was clear my symptoms were just getting worse.

"No," I said. I pressed the nicotine patch a nurse had given to me deeper into the fleshy part of my upper arm. "But when I had benefits through my old job, I saw a private therapist who specialized in dialectical behaviour therapy, which is a treatment for BPD, isn't it?"

"It is. Did you find it helpful?"

I nodded. "Way more than cognitive behavioural therapy."

"Let's take a look at the symptoms of BPD together," Rick said. He pulled a single sheet of paper from the folder that sat on the table between us.

Rick had paid me a compliment about self-awareness while he was on the precipice of suggesting I had one of the hardest-to-treat and least-understood personality disorders on record. I think he was trying to fortify me against what was to come. I would soon take on a label that coloured all of my future interactions with the mental health community. And one that many psychiatrists would simply refuse to treat.

✳

BPD has long confounded the medical community. Adolph Stern was among the first to attempt to define and characterize the disorder. In an obituary published in the *Psychoanalytic Quarterly*, Stern was remembered as a "self-effacing, serene man of astute [and] practical wisdom," who enjoyed playing golf and spent much of his free time talking about psychoanalysis to anyone who would listen, never missing an opportunity to share his knowledge with others. By the time he died at his New Jersey vacation home in 1958, the physician's influence on psychiatry and psychoanalysis had been significant.

Stern was the first American psychoanalyst to train with Sigmund Freud and was one of the few remaining first-generation psychoanalysts in America at the time of his death. He was president of the New York Psychoanalytic Society for three terms. His theories are described in the *History of Countertransference* as "hugely relevant."

As psychoanalysis fell out of favour, Stern was remembered not for his contributions to the Freudian practice but as the so-called father of the psychiatric use of the term *borderline*. In 1938, Stern presented a seminal paper, "Psychoanalytic Investigation of and Therapy in the Border Line Group of Neuroses," to the New York Psychoanalytic Society. In his paper, he chronicled patients who were neither psychotic nor neurotic. It was a group that had been previously described by American physician Irving Rosse in 1890 as "a class of persons standing in the twilight of right reason and despair . . . Individuals with minds trembling in the balance between reason and madness, are not so sane as to be able to control themselves, nor yet so insane as to require restraint or seclusion." Like Rosse, Stern found these people similarly confounding. He noted that "this border line [sic] group of patients is extremely difficult to handle effectively by any psychotherapeutic method." When he tried to treat these people, Stern found psychoanalysis offered little help. More often than not, Stern offered no treatment at all because of poor therapeutic outcomes. But he was encountering more people with the disorder in his practice and believed identifying this group of people was vital in order to successfully treat them.

Before Stern, psychoanalysts considered the disorder an invalid, or wastebasket, concept. The first characteristic of BPD that Stern described was narcissism below the normal range. He noted that the people he deemed borderline had significant deficits in their levels of self-worth and self-assurance, which he proposed resulted from a lack of early affection from caregivers and drove the other symptoms of the disorder. These included "psychic bleeding," or a vulnerability to painful or traumatic experiences, hypersensitivity that could develop into mild paranoia, a lack of tolerance for change, poor responses to treatment, feelings of inferiority, masochism or high rates of self-inflicted harm, anxiety, a tendency to project negative expectations onto the world around the sufferer, and difficulties in thinking realistically or altered perceptions of reality. Stern was instrumental in recognizing the symptoms of what is now understood as BPD. However, the term *borderline* belonged to neither classic psychoanalysis nor traditional psychiatry. Instead, it represented a liminal state for those whose mental health bordered on numerous established diagnoses.

✳

Before 1970, people with BPD were largely seen as extremely difficult to treat or altogether untreatable.

In the 1980s, psychiatry started its shift away from psychoanalysis and into more biological understandings of mental illness. The interdisciplinary approach recognized mental illnesses as a function of the nervous system, which allowed researchers to differentiate BPD from illnesses like schizophrenia or depression. More studies emerged that illuminated the connection between BPD and early traumatic experiences. This paved the way for the rise of non-psychoanalytic treatments for the disorder like cognitive behavioural, group, or family therapy, methods that were more effective.

However, it wasn't until the 1990s—the decade that I arrived in the world—that BPD treatment really advanced. And it wasn't thanks to a white man in a lab coat but to a woman with her own lived experience: Marsha M. Linehan.

Linehan was born in 1943 in Tulsa, Oklahoma, one of six children in a "highly-respected, upper-middle-class family." She was always a bit different from the rest of her household—talkative and curvy in a community and era that expected women to be obedient and slim. In her memoir, *Building a Life Worth Living*, she admitted her childhood nickname was "Million-Ton Motor Mouth."

Linehan lived in a stable environment and didn't experience any significant trauma, but her mother never quite accepted her for who she was. Perhaps this is part of the reason why Linehan entered a depression so severe in her senior year of high school that she wouldn't leave her bedroom. She was admitted to the Institute of Living in Hartford, Connecticut. She spent the next two years in the hospital and received electroconvulsive therapy in addition to being forcibly isolated, medicated, and restrained. Once institutionalized, she displayed many symptoms of BPD—self-harm and suicidal thoughts, volatile mood swings, pervasive feelings of emptiness, impulsive behaviour, dissociation, and frantic efforts to avoid separation from her doctor. Linehan wasn't formally diagnosed with the disorder but concedes her behaviour during inpatient care met the criteria for BPD.

But, like anyone with the disorder, Linehan was so much more than her destructive behaviours or the trauma she experienced while trying to treat them. During her time in Hartford, Linehan made a vow to get herself out of the hell she was experiencing—and to help others in her position do the same thing.

✳

My loved ones had been concerned about my volatile moods since I was a child. I often spent weekends with my Grandma Kath, or G.K., as she's affectionately known even by those outside her family. I remember her, halted while crossing her sun-filled apartment, staring at me intently, like she was scanning a troubling skyline. "Get in the kitchen, Miranda. It's time to make a cake."

Before the medical industry labelled my mood swings as depression, anxiety, PTSD, or BPD, G.K. called them conniption fits. She says she could tell one was coming because my eyes would change. "They'd get darker somehow," she told me years later. In true grandma fashion, her fix wasn't medicine, therapy, or defining what was happening to me. It was baking. The low hum of the electric mixer, the delicate crack of an eggshell splintering on the side of a porcelain bowl, and the wafting scent of vanilla extract could clear the clouds in my eyes.

The more cynical members of my family believed my outbursts were childish manipulations, that I was misbehaving to get my way. When I was eight, my mother brought me to our small-town family doctor in hopes of finding a medical explanation for my fits. I don't remember speaking during the visit—just staring at the doctor's wiry knuckle hair. He frowned while my mother described my symptoms and said they were likely the result of a food sensitivity. Probably to chocolate and the red and yellow dyes used to colour candies; lots of kids had bad reactions to them. He didn't administer an allergy test or refer me to a specialist, but my mother was content with the suggestion because I was high-functioning in so many other aspects of childhood—socially, academically, and creatively. After the doctor's visit, I was largely banished from baking the brownies and polka-dotted pineapple upside-down cakes that proved such an effective distraction (though G.K., always a bit of a brat, occasionally ignored this rule).

My family members weren't the only ones worried about my emotional responses. I was too. I was acutely aware that other children didn't run away from home, tears blowing into the wind, to hide beneath suburban mailboxes or in nearby playgrounds. So, not believing the doctor's allergy explanation, I did what my mother did when my brother or I was sick. I pulled down her medical dictionary, sandwiched between Stephen King books, from the hulking mahogany cabinet it was kept in. It was dense and general. Its pages defined everything from the common cold to leprosy.

I knew my symptoms weren't external. Whatever happened did so inside my mind. What I understood as craziness at that point was limited to media depictions: Bart Simpson being carted off to the madhouse for spotting a gremlin no one else noticed in "Treehouse of Horror IV"; the mad wife of Edward Rochester in a movie adaptation of *Jane Eyre*, locked away in an attic for a decade until she sets the house on fire and flings herself from the roof; or Leela from *Futurama*'s sorrowful but familiar admission that she usually kept her sadness pent up inside where it could "fester quietly as a mental illness." I was left to glean mental health diagnoses from pop culture and cross-reference them with the medical dictionary. I hoped that if I pinpointed what was wrong with me, I might avoid some of the uglier fates that had befallen these characters. A definition might help me better understand my fluctuating moods, the pit of despair lodged in my heart, and why I seemed to create so much friction in my household. It might tell me how to be like everyone else. It might tell me what I had to do in order to heal. I wanted so much to feel better.

Mental health diagnostics is more art than science. It's slippery, like trying to find a pebble in a hailstorm. Had I known then how subjective and inexact an exercise it can be, I might have spent fewer hours poring over the glossy pages of the medical dictionary. But most afternoons, once I had finished my homework for the day, I lugged the tome to our tartan couch, flicked on the television, and skimmed through its pages, searching for an illness that reflected my experience. The closest I ever came was rapid cycling manic depression, now known as a form of bipolar disorder. I saw myself in the mood swings described in the literature, but the duration was wrong. I could cycle through four to six moods over the course of a Michelina's TV dinner. Manic moods were described as lasting much longer. What was clear about my research was that I couldn't ask my family for help. Whatever was wrong with me couldn't be treated with NyQuil or Polysporin. This wasn't like a cold, flu, or that time my brother had whooping cough. It was an illness bound in shame, whispered quietly about by family members, and treated in places where the sufferer was locked away, relegated to a metaphorical attic where the disorder wouldn't trouble healthy loved ones.

Even if I had found BPD in my mother's medical dictionary or had been diagnosed by my family doctor, there were few treatment options available to children in the late 1990s. Prevailing knowledge at the time was that the disorder couldn't be reliably diagnosed in people under eighteen. Diagnosing adolescents with the disorder was considered precarious because so many of BPD's symptoms are common to puberty: emotional instability, identity uncertainty, fears of rejection, and impulsive behaviour. However, like me, many people with BPD experienced symptoms of the disorder as early as childhood. Recent studies have confirmed that BPD can be reliably diagnosed in adolescents as young as eleven years old if the symptoms persist for longer than a year.

Contemporary knowledge of mental health favours early intervention: the sooner a mental illness is treated, the better. A 2008 *British Journal of Psychiatry* randomized trial on a limited sample size showed that early intervention for BPD was not only possible but also resulted in significant positive effects for the adolescents who received it. Early intervention in many mental illnesses, including those influenced by traumatic experiences, can act as a protective factor that improves the long-term trajectory of a person's physical and mental health.

In order to treat a mental health disorder, early or otherwise, it's crucial to understand the illness. But BPD is a historically misunderstood condition. As early as 1953, a borderline diagnosis was applied to people who weren't easy to classify. That year, psychoanalyst Robert P. Knight wrote a bulletin for the Menninger Clinic, a notable psychiatric hospital in Kansas. The bulletin, "Borderline States," expressed frustration that the label, when used as a diagnosis, "conveys more information about the uncertainty and indecision of the psychiatrist than it does about the condition of the patient." The paper was also the first to frame BPD as an enduring personality structure with significant impairments in the mental processes that help people deal with their feelings, thoughts, and reactions. And it hit upon what would become one of the notable characteristics of the disorder: the high rate at which it can be found in treatment settings. Knight's "Borderline States" set the stage for the eventual classification of the illness as a personality disorder.

Two decades later, it was another Menninger Clinic staff member who made important advances in how BPD was understood. Austrian-American psychoanalyst Otto F. Kernberg was described by Linehan as the "kindest of human beings," which is perhaps why he chose to study disorders that were so maligned by the mental health community. He studied people with severe neurotic illnesses and personality disorders. This gave him insight into what he called borderline personality organization, or BPO. People with BPO tended to use "childish" or "extreme" ways of dealing with impulses and emotions, like self-harm or reality denial. They tended to view others as all good or all bad (now known as splitting) and were cognitively more disorganized than most—particularly under stress. Kernberg's concept of BPO influenced the development of the disorder's criteria and interest among the medical professionals who treated it.

Kernberg's work with people with BPD would help influence Linehan's career trajectory. After leaving psychiatric care, Linehan pursued an undergraduate degree in psychology at Loyola University Chicago and graduated as one of the top students in her year. She earned her M.A. there in 1970 and her Ph.D. the following year, focusing on gender differences in suicide. By the time she was hired at the University of Washington in Seattle, her background studying suicide and behavioural therapy inspired her to take on the task of developing an effective treatment for highly suicidal people.

"I target suicidal, out-of-control behaviour," Linehan wrote in her memoir. "I don't think of myself as treating a disorder. I treat a set of behaviours that gets turned into a disorder by others."

Linehan didn't necessarily intend to create a treatment protocol for people with BPD, but to receive funding for her research, she needed to treat a disorder and not a behaviour. The behaviour she tried to treat—chronic suicidality and self-harm—was most often found in people with BPD.

Linehan developed dialectical behavioural therapy (DBT) by incorporating her own lived and professional experience and her accreditation as a Zen master with existing behavioural therapies. DBT focuses on acceptance and change—the opposing therapeutic goals that inspired the dialectical approach of her treatment. The therapy involves group skill-building sessions, one-on-one psychotherapy sessions, phone support, and a clinical consultation team. DBT didn't obey the traditional rules of therapy or take its lead from Kernberg's notoriously rigid treatment of people with the disorder. For example, people in DBT programs were free to call their therapist outside treatment hours.

During the first clinical trial of the treatment, Linehan found that women with BPD who received DBT were far less likely to injure themselves than those who received traditional therapy. But plenty of professionals in the field were extremely skeptical about her results. They insisted her success arose from her competence and not because DBT worked. Linehan, a woman with incredible persistence, conducted sixteen additional randomized trials independently run by a host of therapists. Each trial resulted in the same outcomes as the first. Subsequent research demonstrated that DBT also improved individuals' relationships with themselves and the people responsible for treating them. Kernberg would go on to praise Linehan as the only professional "whose treatment matches the theory on which it's based."

In the sparse hospital meeting room, my grumbling stomach seemed as loud as a roar. It had been six hours since I had arrived at the hospital and longer than that since I'd had a meal. The overhead lights flickered slightly, seeming to shiver with me as I read the symptoms of BPD.

At the top of the piece of paper Rick gave me, the disorder was defined generally as a "pervasive pattern of instability in interpersonal relationships, self-image, and emotion, as well as marked impulsivity beginning by early adulthood and present in a variety of contexts." But it was the symptoms that followed that really resonated with me. I read about people with BPD's frantic efforts to avoid abandonment, their damaging impulsivity, recurrent suicidal behaviour and self-harm, mood swings, chronic feelings of emptiness, tendency to dissociate, and their unstable and intense interpersonal relationships. It was like looking into a mirror. I felt the sense of satisfaction that I experienced when I finished a puzzle, each piece coming together to form a full picture.

But contention and controversy persist around the validity and usefulness of a BPD diagnosis.

In order for me to meet the threshold for a diagnosis, I needed to experience at least five of the nine symptoms from the *Diagnostic and Statistical Manual of Mental Disorders* IV (*DSM-IV*) definition that Rick shared with me. This allows for 256 possible symptom combinations and countless presentations of the disorder. If I did have BPD, it was highly unlikely it would look like someone else's.

The broad nature of the disorder is one of the reasons the National Alliance of Mental Illness considers BPD one of the most misdiagnosed mental illnesses. The wide spectrum of BPD presentations, coupled with the fact that it's a clinical label with no supporting medical tests, often makes it challenging for mental health professionals to diagnose BPD. Clinicians only have a limited amount of time to label the people they're treating in part because mental health care in Canada is sorely underfunded, under-resourced, and separated into a labyrinth of departments even the most determined bureaucrat couldn't untangle.

BPD overlaps with several established diagnoses, another reason why it's frequently misdiagnosed. According to a 2020 *Mental Health Practice* article, people with autism spectrum disorder (ASD) and BPD share challenges in understanding and responding to emotions in themselves and others and display difficulties with social interactions. But ASD is commonly understood as a neurological disorder, whereas BPD tends to be associated with early adverse environmental experiences like childhood abuse or neglect. Self-harm is a prevalent symptom in both disorders but is thought to serve different functions. It tends to occur in people with ASD when they're experiencing sensory overload, and in people with BPD during interpersonal conflict or emotional dysregulation. Various studies have also pointed to co-occurrences of BPD and ASD. A 2017 study found people with BPD had elevated autistic traits and a strong drive to systemize like those with ASD. A 2008 study of a small sample of women with BPD found that 15 per cent of patients also fulfilled the criteria for ASD. There's a notable gender difference between diagnoses: BPD is more often diagnosed in women, and ASD is more often diagnosed in men.

BPD has long been considered a woman's disorder. This is likely due to an oft-repeated statistic that BPD affects women at a rate of three to one. If one looks closely at the data this statistic originates from, they'll find it's based entirely on populations in clinical settings. Therefore, it's more accurate to say women seek help for BPD at three times the rate men do. More recent research suggests BPD is equally prevalent in women and men.

Like I did when I was researching illnesses in my mother's dictionary, medical professionals are known to confuse BPD symptoms with bipolar disorder. There are many crossover traits: elevated suicide rates, functional impairment, and emotional dysregulation. However, bipolar disorder is seen as a disease of the brain; BPD is viewed as a disease of the personality. Bipolar disorder can be effectively controlled and managed through medication, diet, and exercise. While a healthy diet and regular exercise can help reduce vulnerability to moods, extensive therapy is the primary form of treatment for people with BPD. There's also evidence that BPD may be underdiagnosed in favour of bipolar disorder. A 2009 study showed that 40 per cent of people who met the criteria for BPD, but not bipolar disorder, were nonetheless diagnosed with bipolar type II. Many clinicians view BPD as treatment-resistant or are hesitant to diagnose the disorder in people because it's less understood and resourced than bipolar disorder. But this prevents people with BPD from getting the help they actually need and discourages researchers from studying the disorder.

It's also very rare to find cases of "pure BPD." It can co-occur with ASD and bipolar disorder, but it typically exists side by side with depression, anxiety, and substance use disorders, which contributes to misdiagnosis. A 1988 comparative study found that 91 per cent of people with BPD in inpatient settings had at least one additional diagnosis, and 42 per cent had two or more additional diagnoses. More recent studies found that 96 per cent of people with BPD also have a mood disorder. Lifetime depression rates are between 71 and 83 per cent. Eighty-eight per cent of people with BPD have anxiety disorders. People with BPD are also likely to suffer from panic disorder, post-traumatic stress disorder (PTSD), or eating disorders. A small 2020 study from the *European Archives of Psychiatry and Clinical Neuroscience* even suggested that most participants with BPD met the criteria for a schizophrenia spectrum disorder. It's been nearly a century since BPD was first identified as a mental illness that bordered on other established diagnoses, but the disorder hasn't become any less murky.

Perhaps this is why some clinicians—though it remains widely debated—consider BPD a trauma-spectrum disorder. People with BPD tend to experience extremely high rates of early traumatic experiences like neglect or abuse. A 2019 meta-analysis found people with BPD were more than thirteen times more likely to have experienced early trauma than those without a mental illness. And there's a significant overlap between BPD and complex post-traumatic stress disorder (C-PTSD). A 2021 *Frontiers in Psychiatry* review article noted that BPD and C-PTSD share dissociative symptoms, emotional dysregulation, disturbances in relationships, and self-dysregulation. The authors point out that chronic and recurring trauma early in life increases the inability to control emotions, which can result in the behavioural patterns seen in BPD.

I righted the sheet of paper and slid it back across the table to Rick. "I would say I meet all of the symptoms except for intense anger," I said. "Especially the fear of abandonment. I'm always worried that the people I care about are going to leave me. It dictates basically everything I do."

Rick waited for a Code White announcement, a hospital code that indicates a person on the premises is at risk to themselves or others, to finish playing over the PA system. "That's pretty common in people with BPD," he said.

I rubbed my swollen eyelids, which were puffed up like inner tubes from all the crying I'd done on the walk to the hospital. I asked Rick if BPD was a challenging diagnosis. I had heard that there was no medication approved to treat it.

"That's true," Rick said. "But you can take medication to improve the associated symptoms like your depression and anxiety. And understanding of BPD is evolving. Many clinicians see it as a disorder rooted in chronic trauma, closer to post-traumatic stress disorder, which aligns with your history."

I sighed. "Okay. I really don't care what I'm labelled with. I just need some help that will give me relief. I can't keep getting hospitalized. I can't keep feeling this way."

The depression I displayed during my interview with Rick was among the primary symptoms noted by mental health professionals who observed people with BPD. In 1968, the first evidence-based research about the disorder was published. In his book *The Borderline Syndrome*, psychiatrist Roy R. Grinker attempted to classify and quantify the disturbed behaviour found in people with the disorder. He and his colleagues noted four characteristics to better identify people with BPD, including a predominant emotional state of expressed anger, defects in emotional relationships, impairments in self-identity, and depressive loneliness. This observation-based approach to the disorder laid the groundwork for further understanding and clarifying diagnostic features.

Ultimately, it was the combined work of psychiatrists John G. Gunderson and Robert L. Spitzer that led to the recognition of BPD as an official psychiatric diagnosis. In 1975, Gunderson collaborated with clinical psychologist Margaret T. Singer on "Defining Borderline Patients: An Overview." The article reviewed existing research to refine the main characteristics of the disorder and found six features that might allow clinicians to better diagnose people with BPD during an initial interview: an intense depressive or hostile affect, a history of impulsive behaviour, brief psychotic experiences, relationships that swing between dependency and superficiality, some ability to adapt socially, and disorganized thinking in unstructured situations. Gunderson went on to develop the Diagnostic Interview for Borderline Patients, a research instrument that allowed those studying the disorder to more easily identify it and compare findings. Around the time Gunderson and Singer were creating their overview of BPD, Robert Spitzer, an established psychiatrist working on a criteria-based method for assessing and sorting psychiatric symptoms, became the chair of the third edition of the *DSM*, a reference book that's now viewed as psychiatry's bible. It was this edition that drastically changed the field of psychology. It transformed the manual from a text that gathered dust on doctors' shelves to a book that was exalted for standardizing psychiatric diagnoses. Spitzer led the charge to create distinct diagnostic categories across mental illnesses, including a five-part diagnostic system, which is still used today.

Spitzer formed working groups of clinical experts on various disorders, including BPD, over deli lunches in cramped meeting rooms. He created potential criteria for the disorder, based largely on the work Gunderson and Singer completed, which was evaluated by a group of psychiatrists from across the United States. The resulting set of characteristics became the basis for BPD.

How BPD was understood had evolved significantly in the forty years since Stern coined the term to its appearance in the *DSM-III*. But the arbitrary name for the disorder stuck.

✳

Just as understanding of the disorder has evolved, so have treatment options. Since Linehan published her first randomized trial about

DBT, over thirteen different psychotherapies for BPD have been tested and four have been established as evidence-based treatments. Transference-focused therapy, based on Kernberg's object relations theory, helps people with BPD heal their problematic behaviour by exploring it through the person-therapist relationship. Schema-focused therapy was developed by Jeffrey E. Young to treat personality disorders by reshaping unhealthy coping patterns. In 1995, systems training for emotional predictability and problem-solving (STEPPS) was created by Nancee S. Blum. STEPPS is a group treatment meant to complement ongoing individual therapies by teaching people with BPD how to identify, change, and manage behaviours and feelings that come with the disorder. In the late 1990s, Peter Fonagy and Anthony Bateman developed mentalization-based treatment, which helps people with BPD develop the skills they need to attend to the mental states of themselves and others before reacting.

Linehan had kept her promise. She had gotten herself and countless others out of the hell they were experiencing. And she had inspired new treatments to help the people who were left behind. But she kept her mental health history (and her scars from self-injury) carefully hidden throughout her professional career. In 2011, she returned to the Institute of Living to deliver a speech. At sixty-eight years old, motivated by the people she treated, Linehan told the world her whole story.

"So many people have begged me to come forward, and I just thought—well, I have to do this. I owe it to them. I cannot die a coward," Linehan told *The New York Times* a week after she had made her mental health history public.

✷

"I think we should keep you on a short-term hold in emergency admitting while you feel you're a danger to yourself. And then we can connect you to inpatient or outpatient services for BPD. How does that sound?" Rick asked.

"Okay."

I was finally through the admitting process. Back in the waiting room, I updated my partner, gave him a lingering hug, and pulled the strap of the overnight bag we'd packed for the occasion onto my shoulder.

I was led through locked glass doors to a dreary room with two beds, both unoccupied. The lone window looked out onto dying clumps of weeds and a fence that sectioned off an electrical box. I had been allowed to keep some notebooks and a deck of cards, but the rest of my possessions were up at the nurses' station, which served as the focal point of the emergency ward. I sat on a bed and began to deal myself into a game of solitaire when a shrill scream penetrated the wall nearest to me. I jerked in surprise.

"Where am I?" a disembodied voice from the room next to mine asked. It began to whimper. Then scream. "What's going on? Why am I here?"

I sighed. Definitely not the most calming place to heal from my suicidal urges. But if I could stick it out, maybe I'd finally address some of the root causes of my difficulties instead of just treating the symptoms.

✷

So, why do I choose to identify with such a poorly understood and frequently maligned disorder—particularly when people with BPD are known for their sensitivity to rejection? Living with BPD is intense. The word *borderline*, when used as a noun, means a division between two distinct and often extreme conditions. It evokes an image of an individual poised between opposing states; however, people with BPD rarely find that balance. Instead, we lead a life of extremes in a society that tells us moderation is the secret ingredient to good health. We ping-pong between emotions like anger and happiness, paranoia and hope, rage and inertia. These feelings are overwhelming, painful, and hard to control—emotions so strong it feels like our blood is boiling. We become the emotion. Researchers call this state "the affective storm of BPD." The disorder is often compared to weather events for its unpredictability and the powerlessness that the people who support us feel in the face of it. Like many serious mental illnesses, BPD is a disorder in which more attention is paid to how we affect the people around us than how the symptoms affect us.

As more straightforward diagnoses like depression and anxiety shed the shame that used to come with the illnesses, BPD remains in the shadows with other "scary" labels like schizophrenia or bipolar disorder. But living with the illness isn't just terror and torment. People with BPD can be highly intelligent and creative. Timely studies show we have enhanced empathetic abilities and have talent in involving and influencing others. We feel intensely and love intensely. BPD can look like an extreme lack of emotional intelligence, but that gives me hope—hope that I can learn to live with the disorder better. And help others through my experience. There is plenty written about how excruciating and terrifying it is to live with BPD (and there will be glimpses of that in the book you're holding), but it's not all bad. And neither are we. I emphasize *people with* BPD in this book and not *borderlines* or BPD *patients*, because that's what we are—people before anything else. We're human beings with many gifts and positive attributes who are labelled with a broad disorder because we have trouble moving through the world in a way that's considered familiar or normal—behaviours that were never modelled to us when we were growing up.

And maybe if we step into the light, people without the disorder will finally see that.

"How are you feeling this morning?" Rick sat on the foot of my hospital bed.

I stifled a yawn. A woman with dark eyeliner and freckles had been moved into the room's free bed last night. Even if we hadn't spent hours fighting off the effects of our evening meds to compare diagnoses, fretting over whether we had been formed (detained in the hospital until a doctor deemed us fit for release), and discussing which silo of the fragmented mental health system we might end up in, we probably wouldn't have slept anyway. The person in the room next to ours woke up every three hours or so to cry, scream, and ask to go home.

"I'm okay," I said. "Feeling a little hopeful, I guess. I spent so many years in and out of therapy and the hospital without making much progress toward healing. Maybe treatments for BPD and PTSD will be more helpful."

The woman sat on the next bed playing with the deck of cards I had gifted her. She had offered to leave when Rick came in, but I told her not to bother. Privacy on the ward is an illusion.

"That's what we're hoping for," Rick said. "So, you don't feel like you're a risk to yourself right now?"

I shook my head. "There's a light at the end of the tunnel that wasn't there before I came to the hospital."

Rick smiled. "That's great to hear." He scribbled a few notes into a folder and capped his pen. "We have two options going forward. We can discharge you to our outpatient clinic, where we'll get you some short-term counselling and make sure you're put into a DBT skills group. Or we can transfer you upstairs to the women's inpatient floor when a bed becomes available, where you'll also start one-on-one therapy and treatment for BPD and trauma. Based on our conversations, I'm comfortable with either option, so it's up to you."

"How long until a bed becomes available?"

"That's hard to say," Rick said. "You'd stay here in the meantime. And be re-evaluated every twenty-four hours."

"Could I get privileges if I stay? I could really use a smoke."

"Not until you get to the women's ward. This is just the emergency admitting department."

"Hmm." I cupped my chin with my palm. Just then, the person in the next room began yelling again. Rick and I winced at each other.

"Let's do outpatient," I said. And so began my journey along the borderline.

THE BAD GIRLS' SCHOOL

Deep within the unvaried suburbs of Southern Ontario, a six-year-old child stood in front of her bedroom mirror. A pink terrycloth housecoat belt was draped around her neck like a tie waiting to be wrestled into a Windsor knot. The tiny hairs on her nape bristled against the belt's soft fibres when her parents' angry voices strained through her bedroom door, wedged shut with a chair so old its white paint peeled away from the wood. Plump tears marched one by one down her baby-fat cheeks. Shoulders slumped, the girl was overcome. A danger to herself.

The colour pink was synonymous with girlhood in the Western world during the nineties. The shade varied, but it was splashed on everything. Piggy-pink Polly Pockets, hot-pink Barbie convertibles, magenta Doodle Bears to match orchid-pink walls. The colour was inescapable—a visual representation of the innocence that young girls were supposed to embody.

My mother was seduced by the colour. She covered my daybed with a pink-and-white comforter. She stencilled and painted a border of roses to crown the pink walls of my room. She let me wear, almost exclusively, a pink Minnie Mouse dress with a tulle tutu that

I'd eventually throw up on and destroy. The acid from my stomach melted the delicate fabric.

I tried to be more careful when I was gifted a pink housecoat. In the mornings, my mother mutely drifted through the halls of our house in her own pink housecoat, steaming coffee in hand. I trailed behind her. Two females moved through the dawn's shadows in matching robes. I watched her prepare for her day, following her into the bathroom, where she'd light a cigarette, its smoke curling up into the noisy fan, slough off her housecoat, and fill the tub. She always sighed when she sank into the warm water. Her floating breasts were two pink mountains surrounded by clouds of soapy suds.

The Madonna of the Pinks, a painting by Raphael, is small enough to fit in the palm of a hand. Displayed in London's National Gallery, an ocean away, I've only seen it online. The painting shows the Virgin Mary in a darkened room. She's dressed in muted greens and cerulean blue, handing a flower to the infant Christ, who sits upon a white pillow in her lap. The flower, a pink carnation, is said by the gallery to represent "divine love and was reputed to have sprung from the earth where the Virgin's tears fell during Christ's Passion." A godless girl, raised by a woman whose personal Madonna sang "Papa Don't Preach," I tend to favour the secular interpretation of the carnation's meaning: that the flower symbolizes friendship and betrothal or the spiritual marriage between mother and child (still theologically appropriate as Mary was referred to as both the bride and mother of Christ). Raphael is well-known for his Madonnas. His depictions of mother and child are touchingly tender, imbued with a hushed gentleness that reveals the profound bond the two share. In *The Madonna of the Pinks*, it's the delicate pink blossom of the divine flower, so easily crushed by a closed palm, that communicates the sacred union.

But what about the paternal bond? There are only hints of a masculine presence in Raphael's painting. The draped bed the Virgin sits near is said to signify the green wedding bed from biblical texts. Neither Mary nor Christ seems bothered by the physical lack of a father, content to peacefully delight in each other's company. I imagine they don't even register his absence, the same way my own absent father had no influence on me when I followed my mother's billowing pink housecoat from room to room, content to delight in her quiet tenderness.

In the first photograph, I'd guess I'm not yet a year old. At the bottom of my warm and trusting smile, two baby teeth that glisten with drool are emerging from pink gums. My eyes haven't yet lost their blue. A frilled sock hangs from my small foot, which rests next to the plastic wheel of a Fisher-Price telephone with eyes that rolled up and down when you pushed it. My gaze is directed up and to the right of the camera lens, where I imagine my mother was standing, cooing encouragement, asking me to say "cheese" for the photographer. There's an air of confusion about my brow like I'm not quite sure why I've been brought to this bright room to sit primly in my floral dress in front of a stranger. But my gaze is trusting and filled with love. I'm safe with my mother, who might be playing peekaboo with me, her slender hands cupped in front of her glasses, or grinning as wide as she can, her mouth modelling what she hoped I would mimic.

The second photo is from junior kindergarten. I was four years old. My stepdad had moved in the year before. Giant magenta roses bloom across my turtleneck tracksuit. My bangs are cut in a sharp line across my forehead. I sit awkwardly in a white wicker chair. My shoulders are tense and pulled up to the bottom of my ears. My left hand death-grips the top of my right, which turns the tips of my fingers white. My lips are unsmiling. The top lip is chapped. Dying skin is visible beneath the cupid's bow. The bottom is red and swollen. The patch of skin beneath is so inflamed it erases the borderline between flesh and lip. I remember my lips felt like sandpaper, so dry that I kept licking them, only aggravating the discomfort. My eyes, green filling in around the pupil, stare beyond the lens far off into some distant place. Vacant. Fearful.

✳

In 1977, Louise Kapp Howe, a writer who specialized in social issues, published *Pink Collar Workers: Inside the World of Women's Work*. Nominated for a National Book Award, it highlighted the ways in which the workforce was still segregated and trapped women in low-paying care-oriented jobs like child education, hospitality, or retail. It also popularized the term *pink-collar worker*. Housewives and women who chose to stay at home with their children were included in Howe's read on the pink-collar workforce, a novel addition that demonstrated how a woman's role as a homemaker can interfere with her occupational success.

In a 1993 study published in *Industrial Relations*, author Gerald Hunt compared men's and women's experiences in the pink-collar workforce. Men who were surveyed were more likely to find their work trivial and tedious. They were also less committed to their pink-collar roles. Many emphasized that it was merely a stable paycheque that allowed them to achieve creative pursuits like writing or music. Or it was a way to avoid the pressures of more male-dominated fields. For men, pink work was meant to be temporary. A transient role until something more worthwhile came along.

※

"Bad girl, bad girl, whatcha gonna do? Whatcha gonna do when they come for you?" My stepdad liked to taunt me with the theme song from *Cops*, a grungy reality show that followed police officers as they tormented people who lived far beneath the poverty line.

It was possible he sang it while I was shadowed in the kitchen of our small townhouse, my four-year-old fingers prodding the haired skin inside my nostrils, hoping to dislodge a booger. He was splayed on the couch in front of the television in ratty boxer shorts. It was his preferred spot for whiling away the extended hours before my mother returned from work to help care for me and my infant brother.

"You better not be picking your nose in there," he yelled. His tone was sharp and angry, but his words were sticky and slurred by

Percocet or OxyContin or whatever opioid his doctor had prescribed to erase his pain from a car accident he'd been in before he
crash-landed into my life. His pelvis had shattered, splintered into
as many fragments as the windshield he flew headfirst through and
the tree trunk his pickup truck slammed into. Unable to work his
blue-collar union job, he was placed on disability. He was paid to
stay home. To play Mr. Mom. But, like the men surveyed about
their experiences in pink-collar roles, my stepdad found the work
trivial and tedious. It was a transient role meant merely to fill the
hours until my mom came home.

My stepdad stomped into the kitchen. I froze. A small pink finger was stuck in my left nostril. His eyes blazed wildly. His tobacco-
stained teeth emerged from his sneer. My heart pounded loudly in
my ears. I bolted like a criminal hunted down by a wash of red-and-
blue sirens. His footsteps thundered behind me. I willed my burning
legs to go faster, up the stairs, and into the safety of my bedroom. I
slammed the door to my room shut, placed two hands against the
smooth wood, and leaned my full body weight into it. My breath
escaped my mouth in small sharp bursts. He was swearing in the
hallway. I heard the crash and felt the door lurch in its frame before
I noticed I was airborne. I slammed into the wall behind me. Hot
pain filled the shoulder that absorbed the impact.

I was yanked down the carpeted staircase, my injured shoulder
painfully straining in its socket. My feet stumbled and scraped the
stairs, but my stepdad's grip kept me aloft. The walls of our townhouse were blurred by my tears. I sobbed while I put on my shoes,
securing the Velcro straps; my little fingers had yet to figure out how

to tie laces. The front door slammed behind us and echoed through the cul-de-sac. My stepdad pulled me into the crimson maw of his hulking black truck. "I've had it up to here," he said while he strapped me into my booster seat. "I'm taking you to the Bad Girls' School."

My one-year-old brother must've been with us. Surely, he wouldn't have been left to play with his toys on the living room floor. But I only remember wailing in the passenger seat as the truck roared past overgrown lawns and rusty swing sets. The afternoon sun was falling from the top of the sky to paint the corners of dreary strip malls in a menacing pall. I tried to memorize the twists and turns the vehicle made so I might find my way back home.

"You're gonna be real sorry you didn't smarten up when you had the chance," my stepdad said. "The teachers at the Bad Girls' School aren't as nice as I am. They'll hit you with belts and tie you to the bed when you're bad." He told me that little girls who went to the Bad Girls' School weren't allowed to brush their teeth or wash their hair. They ate milky gruel for every meal. And they never saw their mothers.

We screeched to a stop in an empty parking lot. A red brick building loomed over the asphalt. Its windows reflected the day's dwindling glare. Saplings stood motionless beside an abandoned playground.

"We're here," he said. "This is it. The Bad Girls' School."

I sank down into my seat. My shoulder throbbed. I didn't know that the building was just a neighbourhood elementary school. I swore I could feel the eyes of filthy hidden girls boring into the truck's interior.

"Please. I promise I won't ever pick my nose again," I said. An unseen branch cracked in the distance. The bad girls were waiting for me.

"Get out," he said. He reached across me and shoved open the passenger side door.

✳

Childhood always comes with some element of pain: scraped knees, goose eggs, bloody noses, broken bones encased in casts decorated with signatures and well wishes, gravel embedded into road-torn palms, stitches for wounds that won't coagulate, chest infections, sore throats, pink eye. Scars that stay into adulthood. Badges of accomplishment. The price a child pays to navigate the world.

The day I paid my strangest price, I remember the fluttering pink of the inside of my eyelids illuminated by bright hospital lights and weighty from the cough syrup my mother had given me. I had screwed my eyes shut to escape the intrusive stares of my mother, stepfather, and the doctors and nurses in medical scrubs. I was on my back on the exam table. My legs were spread wide. My underwear was off. A nurse told me to take a breath, placed a gentle hand on my round belly, and slipped a tube into my troubled urethra. I gasped. My eyes snapped open. Warm tears fell down the sides of my face.

The procedure was called a cystoscopy. Before we took the dark screeching subway into the city, my mother told me that doctors at a special hospital for sick children needed to look inside my bladder to see why it hurt so much when I peed—why I kept getting infections down there, in that pink private place that strangers weren't supposed to touch.

With the tube inside me, the nurse took my hand and helped me down from the exam table. I walked behind her gingerly, whimpering, stinging inside. She led me to a toilet spotlighted in the centre of the room. It was surrounded by beeping grey machines and a snake pit of wires. Everyone watched me trying to pee. My hospital gown was bunched around my little waist. My feet swung. My legs were too short to reach the tiled floor below.

My thighs shook. My palms grew clammy. Beads of sweat formed across my brow. I pushed so hard that I was either going to go to the bathroom or squeeze out the red-hot invader inside me. I didn't care. Anything to stop the burning.

The pain seethed. A few drops of urine moved through me. The nurse watching said I did good and that we were finished. That the tube could come out.

The hospital never found anything physical to explain my bladder infections. It could be a sensitivity to bubble baths, they suggested. I was banned from my sudsy playtime. No more bubble beards or cloud-like icebergs for my tub toys to navigate.

I never told anyone that I was intentionally holding my pee. The bodily function was the one area of my young life that I could exercise some form of control over. I couldn't change who my mother married or how my stepdad acted. I could choose when I went to the bathroom.

But children's bladders work best when they're emptied on a regular basis. When a child holds their pee, they're more likely to develop UTIs, which make it more painful for them to use the bathroom when they really need to.

I didn't mind pain's fiery lick when it was consistent and reliable. It was the unexpected smacks, the unpredictable screaming, the sudden appearance of snarling rage, the shaking, the hitting, and getting shoved down the stairs that really hurt.

By the time I was in senior kindergarten, we had moved to a bigger house in Bowmanville, a sleepy town east of Toronto. The grey afternoon leaked little light into the living room. My stepdad had lifted my small body so it was eye level with his snapping yellowed teeth.

"I'm going to throw you through the fucking window," he yelled. He shook me by my armpits. His grasp was so powerful that I lost my breath. I feared my delicate rib cage would snap in his hands.

He screamed a resentful cry and hurled me away from his body. The instant I was airborne, I screwed my eyes shut. I imagined I was a ghost, floating beyond the living room, through the shingled roof until I was so high up that our house was indistinguishable from the rest of the subdivision. I braced for the sound of the window's glass cracking across my back like spring ice on a pond. But I must've been heavier than my stepdad anticipated. Or maybe his words were simply a threat to scare me. My small body crashed onto the scratchy couch instead.

My classmates and I learned the basics of colour theory in our vibrant kindergarten classroom, which was papered with our artwork. Primary colours—red, blue, and yellow—were bold powerful shades that couldn't be created by mixing other colours. Instead, they formed secondary colours. Red could be mixed with blue to create purple; yellow and blue combined made green; red and yellow made orange. The colours became darker when we blended any of these hues with our black water-based paint. Adding white produced a lighter version of each shade: lavender, light green, pale orange, and so on.

Except for red. When I smashed the dark bristles of my paintbrush into blood-red paint and combined it with bone white, it made a new colour. Pink. Blood and bone made pink.

I looped the housecoat belt into a simple knot. My emotions felt more painful than my insides that day at the hospital. By trying to anticipate and avoid my stepdad's dark moods, I had warped into a version of myself I no longer recognized. I was like a baby doll zapped in a microwave. I listened for footsteps outside my door. I knew what I was about to do was bad. Dangerous. But no one was coming to check on me. My parents were downstairs and preoccupied, their voices making aggressive crescendos mid-fight. Even if they had checked on me, I didn't have the language skills necessary to communicate the shocking depths of my emotions and convictions. I was still learning how to read.

My act was inspired by the stories of two children who had accidentally strangled themselves with their toys. One was a story I had seen in a made-for-TV movie. The other came from my mother, who had scoured my room for danger after she learned on the radio that a girl had choked to death when she became tangled in a toy hammock. If strangling was lethal for those kids, I reasoned, maybe it was an escape from my frightening stepdad, my tormented emotions, my certainty that I was a very bad girl who could only cause chaos. Maybe it was the solution to my problems.

I gripped each end of the pink belt with chubby fists and pulled as hard as I could. In the mirror's reflection, my face was flushed with blood. My breath wheezed through my constricted throat— a junior version of the death rattle I was ready to embrace. I wanted to die. I gagged and choked. My breath tried to escape the pressure that the knot at the base of my throat created. My red face deepened into a bruised purple. My shining green eyes filled with shock. My vision split into dancing sparkles and blackness. Panicked, my hands, as if acting of their own accord, clawed at the knotted belt and tore it free.

My figure reappeared in my mirror. My chest heaved. The blood slowly drained from my tear-streaked face, turning it back into a fleshy pink. I curled into the fetal position. My cheek rested against rough carpet fibres. A swell of failure and loneliness washed over me. Through the floor, I heard warbled curse words and my mother's sobs.

✳

Baker-Miller pink, also known as P-618 or drunk-tank pink, is a colour used to calm violent, hostile, and aggressive people in institutions.

The shade was discovered by Alexander Schauss, who was a director at the American Institute for Biosocial Research. In the late 1960s, Schauss became interested in the physiological effects of colours on humans while studying at the University of New Mexico. He experimented with colours and noted that when he stared at an eighteen-by-twenty-four-inch card in a specific shade of pink after intense physical exercise his heart rate, pulse, and blood pressure lowered significantly.

Schauss tested hundreds of shades of pink and finally found one that had the greatest effect on reducing excitability: P-618. Schauss then suggested painting the seclusion room at the naval correction centre in Seattle, Washington, with P-618. No incidents of erratic or hostile behaviour occurred in the Baker-Miller pink cell during the 156 days the study took place. The results were replicated at Johns Hopkins University Hospital in Baltimore, Maryland, where researchers learned that the shade can also act as an appetite suppressant. In the following years, Baker-Miller pink was used in prisons, drunk tanks, and psychiatric hospitals with similar success.

A subsequent study conducted on the effects of Baker-Miller pink yielded contradictory results. In 1979, the Santa Clara County Sheriff's Department strip search room was painted pink, but researchers found that aggressive incidents actually increased after the room had been painted for a month. The study hypothesized that perhaps any fresh coat of paint might help minimize violent behaviours in volatile settings.

Maybe finding calm in volatility was why I always selected a shade that, to my untrained eye, resembled Baker-Miller pink when my mother asked what colour I wanted to paint my room. In each new home, I waited patiently while my mother's hands transformed the room that was to be mine from its former life as a little boy's room, sitting area, or, in one instance, a second-floor laundry room. When it was finished, I stepped across the threshold, sighing, comforted by the familiar shade in the strange space. I let the pink walls embrace me.

The reason we moved seemed to change with each dwelling. I knew my mother and I left the first apartment we'd shared after she caught a cockroach strutting across my pink fluffy child-sized armchair. But after that, I can't say. Were we trying to dodge the insurance company surveillance men who sat slumped low in their car across from our townhome, their eyes covered by dark sunglasses when they weren't snapping shots of my stepdad in hopes they might get photographic evidence that he was lying about the extent of his injuries? Or were we trying to find the optimal suburb from which my mother could commute to work so she wasn't so exhausted, her shoulders sagging, a weary forced smile spread thin across her face when she came through the door each night? Was it a simple matter of keeping up with the neighbours? Did my stepdad want to provide a lavish lifestyle for his family regardless of the limits of our bank account?

My stepdad's low moods were terrifying, and his highs were deeply confusing. He had unpredictable moments of generosity, earnestness, and humour that were difficult to reconcile with his sharp words, rough hands, and threats to enforce a code of silence borrowed and bastardized from his Sicilian ancestors. Sometimes he seemed to care: he insisted I call him Dad and offered to legally adopt me—an offer my mother declined. If something happened to her, she wanted me raised by my guardians, her father and her sister. He outfitted the tumbledown cottage his grandmother bought him with snowmobiles, fishing rods, a boat, and a trampoline for me and my brother. He took us on surprise trips to Toys "R" Us and let us choose whatever we wanted from the infinite shelves of glossy boxes. Once, I chose a police officer Barbie, sleek in a black uniform, posed with a smile in front of a backdrop of hot-pink cardboard. I trotted through a few aisles until I found my stepdad and held the shiny box aloft. He smiled. "Throw it in the cart, Da," he said, using the nickname my brother had coined as a toddler when my full name proved too hard to pronounce. His debit card beeped in the machine at the register and scolded us. Insufficient funds. "Better put it back on the shelf," he told me. "We'll get it next time." I had a suspicion when I looked up at my stepdad, shrugging with a grin at the cashier, that I'd never have that doll. When I reminded him of it next time, he scowled and hunched over the shopping cart. "Quit your whining. You have way too many toys as it is—don't even play with half of them."

My stepdad often had good intentions but possessed little foresight. The toys and houses he splurged on were financed by money my maternal grandparents had set aside for my education (which I never saw repaid) and loans from both sides of the family. In the years that followed, we lost almost everything.

Maybe the reasons why we moved so often lurked at a more subconscious and intuitive level. In the tumultuous days of my early childhood, each move was followed by a period of peace. A settling-in. Maybe we needed a fresh coat of paint every so often to placate us. To make us believe that a new environment was going to make us a better and happier family.

✳

"So, you think I'm an asshole, eh? A real prick you wish would just fuck off?" my stepdad asked. My diary sat open on the cottage's coffee table between us. It was a slick laminated number with pink and purple butterflies on the cover.

I had started writing down my thoughts when I was around ten years old after Shirley, an older lady who cottaged across from us, pulled a stack of identical notebooks from her cupboard. We had listened to Doris Day and flipped through forty years of comings and goings, weather reports, animal sightings, cribbage tournament winners, and descriptions of her sons becoming men and fathers. Soon after, Shirley gave me a diary with a lock. There was an illustration of two ballet dancers on the cover. Dressed in a white feathered costume, Odette was clasped in the arms of Siegfried next to the lake they die in during the final act of *Swan Lake*. I filled its pages with daily happenings: the time I flew over the handlebars of the bike with broken rear brakes that my stepdad found at the dump, the time my brother stuffed two dozen frogs down his swimming trunks to win our game of escalating stunts, the time a friend came to stay at the cottage and got homesick—a weakness I couldn't understand or relate to.

But this new diary didn't have a lock. Just glossy pages filled with prompts meant to provoke sentiment. The new diary asked questions like, "When are you happiest at home?" or "Who do you really dislike?" Questions that let emotion drip in like teardrops on a blank page.

"What kind of fucked-up person thinks this way about their family?" my stepdad asked. He gestured to the diary's innards. "There's something seriously wrong with you."

From the grey recliner I sat in, I hugged my knees up to my chest to protect my heart. I castigated myself for being so stupid while my stepdad's reprimands played like a soundtrack in the background. Even if the new diary had had a lock, it's not like it would've kept my feelings safe. Nothing in our house was private, safe, or mine. I knew that. I used to keep my carefully counted quarters, nickels, dimes, and crisp bills from birthdays, Christmases, and babysitting gigs secure inside a red treasure chest fitted with a luggage lock. The flat silver key dangled from a chain I kept around my neck at all times to keep it safe from my stepdad's sticky fingers. I returned from school one afternoon and opened my closet door to find the lock smashed. Broken. A corpse on the carpet. My treasure chest had been emptied. All that remained was a piece of lined paper that listed its pilfered contents (over two hundred dollars) and a sandwich bag of pennies that my stepdad didn't think was worth taking.

"You think you can do and say whatever pops into your head. You never stop to think," my stepdad continued. "And your mother—she just lets you get away with it."

"I'm sorry."

"*Sorry*'s just a word. Doesn't mean shit if you keep making the same mistakes over and over again."

"I know." I scratched at the hem of my jean shorts. I knew it didn't matter what I said. That the punishment wouldn't be over until it was over. That I had hours of humiliation, sarcastic comments, and ego-destroying insults to endure. But maybe if I engrossed myself deep enough into the criss-cross stitchwork, the delicate threads holding my clothes together, I could reduce the discipline's potency to ambient noise.

That night, I crept down to the firepit in the darkness. The flames had dwindled into pulsating embers. The burned wood was ashy. The colour of bone. I tossed the laminated diary into the middle of the pit and watched a column of smoke snake skyward. The pages smouldered and glowed red. Licks of candle-sized flame appeared, danced together, and grew larger. The fire consumed the curling pages until the diary was as ashen as the branches around it. It was the last diary I kept during my childhood.

✳

The winter sun was setting. The sky was a dusky pink. My brother and I sat in separate snow mounds in front of our elementary school. I had collapsed into mine. My eyes were puffy and red from working myself into a flurry of frustrations. My brother was placid. He built snowmen with the mounds of wet packing snow surrounding him.

I heard the crunch of footsteps behind us. "What are you guys still doing here?" The principal blew frosty breath into his naked palms and rubbed them together. "It's pretty cold out."

My brother glanced at the principal and then turned wordlessly back to his snow sculptures.

"We're fine," I said, even though I craved the sound of our truck's auto-locks and the thawing hum of its heater.

The principal had stopped in the tracks his boots made. Clouds of confusion gathered across the horizon of his face. "Really? I see you two waiting out here often. Are you sure I can't call someone for you?"

My brother stopped stacking snowballs to eye me. He lifted an eyebrow—his way of asking if I was going to risk the swearing and rage that came whenever I embarrassed my stepdad by calling home when he was late to pick us up.

"No, thank you," I said.

The principal visibly shivered and hugged his arms to his chest. "Well, why don't we go back inside where it's warm? I can stay with you until your ride gets here."

I knew that warmth came with a price. That if we followed the principal into the school, there would be questions to answer. Questions I couldn't answer without producing a tempest at home.

"No, thank you," I said. "We're fine. I'm sure our dad will be along any minute."

"Are you sure?" The principal glanced between me and my brother.

I nodded. The principal trudged through the slush to his car. I watched his tail lights glow like embers. His worried eyes were framed in the rear-view mirror. He idled in the parking lot for another twenty minutes or so. Finally, he shifted into reverse and his car sighed away from the school.

Fluffy snowflakes floated in the air. The street lights flickered on. I turtled into my winter coat so it pushed up over my lips and warmed the bottom half of my face.

My stepdad's truck slid into the parking lot a little after five. "Sorry, guys," he called out of the passenger-side door. "The clock stopped working. It said it was only three. Can you believe that?" Based on the sleep stuck in the corners of his eyes, I couldn't.

✳

Back in the fourteenth century, *to pink* meant to decorate something with a perforated or punched pattern. Or, more simply, to pierce, stab, or make holes in. At the time, the verb mostly applied to garments.

But isn't this what childhood trauma does? Takes something whole and complete and punches and perforates it until it's warped beyond recognition? Trauma also makes a pattern—a pattern of thoughts, actions, and behaviours that occur as a result of experiences that leave a person forever altered.

Like a piece of fabric sheared with pinking scissors, a traumatized person will never again take the shape they had before they were interfered with. They can only hope the right hands will guide their form into something beautiful. Something complete.

✳

"Let's go back to that little girl with the pink housecoat belt around her neck," my therapist said. We were in her eleventh-floor office in downtown Toronto. The chairs were surprisingly comfortable for publicly covered health care, clearly pilfered over years of careful surveillance and subterfuge.

For as long as I'd been out of my parents' house, about fourteen years by my twenty-ninth birthday, I'd been in and out of therapy.

Many professional hands had tampered with me, grown frustrated, or felt their work was done and left me unfinished, my threads dangling. This particular therapist, undaunted by my borderline personality disorder diagnosis, was trying to braid the strands of my psyche back together using internal family systems therapy, a psychotherapeutic treatment that targets trauma.

I was also working hard to heal, to suture my perforations to a state where I could hold down a job, enjoy my relationship, or take care of myself without splitting apart at the seams. But I still owned that mirror from my childhood. There were many days I stood in front of it, watched my reflection, and felt the same pain I felt when I was six years old. The temptation to die felt woven into me.

Of course, one of the symptoms of BPD is suicidal behaviour, gestures, threats, or self-harm. I had memorized all of the symptoms, read any book that dealt with trauma, and researched the causes of the disorder. My early experiences had taught me that the best way to endure an enemy was to know it well enough that I could anticipate its patterns. And my fractured treatment history demonstrated that it was largely left up to me to do the necessary reconnaissance. I started where anyone would. At the beginning. With the causes of the disorder.

I read about John Bowlby, the British psychiatrist who pioneered attachment theory. As in many upper-middle-class families in England in the early twentieth century, Bowlby spent little time with his mother or father as a child and was mainly brought up by nannies. As an adult, he believed the emotional disturbances he witnessed in the maladjusted children he worked with were caused by their family circumstances. Attachment theory posits that infants develop close emotional bonds with their caregivers instinctively for survival, safety, and social and emotional development. Bowlby noted that infants who were separated from their parents would cry, cling, or search to provoke a reunion with their missing caregiver. He hypothesized that the attachment behaviours he witnessed were adaptive responses. Children who stayed physically close to their caretakers were more likely to survive to maturity. Natural selection favoured a behavioural motivation system that encouraged a child's proximity to their parent.

In 1950, Mary Salter Ainsworth, a Canadian-American developmental psychologist, studied Bowlby's theories under laboratory conditions. Ainsworth observed three distinct attachment styles in the toddlers she studied, though a fourth was added later to fit infant behaviour that she found difficult to classify—or, in other words, behaviour that bordered on numerous attachment styles. Children who used their caregiver as a safe base from which to explore the world were considered securely attached. Children who showed little interest in their caregiver, had a history of not having their needs met, and were thought to stay close enough to their caregivers to feel protected but distant enough to avoid rejection had an avoidant or anxious insecure attachment style. Children who were more distressed and less likely to explore their environment, a sign of inconsistent or unpredictable caregiving, had an ambivalent or resistant insecure attachment style. The fourth group of children displayed odd, inexplicable, or conflicted behaviours toward their caregivers. These children often came from abusive and unpredictable environments, had parents who were dealing with unresolved traumas, or were parented by adults who had formed insecure attachments with their own caregivers. Children from the fourth group had a disorganized or disoriented insecure attachment style. Unresolved attachment is strongly associated with BPD. One study found that as many as 92 per cent of people with the disorder displayed insecure attachment patterns, especially anxious or disorganized styles. Each attachment style correlated with a unique presentation of the disorder in adulthood. People with BPD who had an avoidant attachment style with their caregivers couldn't regulate their emotions because no one had taught them how to. When they failed to regulate their emotions, they engaged in impulsive behaviours. People with BPD who had an anxious attachment style were unable to manage their anxiety as adults. They were easily overwhelmed. Lacking healthy emotional regulation skills, they were likely to quiet these feelings through self-harm or reckless behaviour. Disorganized attachment styles, particularly in circumstances where there was abuse or neglect, resulted in adults with BPD who experienced dissociation, hallucinations, and personality disturbances.

It's difficult to retroactively identify my attachment style. My behaviour aligns with numerous unresolved attachment types. I know what it's like to act before I think. To find myself in dangerous situations. To feel so overwhelmed it was as if there was an air raid siren inside my head and the only logical way to silence it was to destroy myself. I know what it's like to be unable to express anger because I associated the emotion with my stepdad's violence, and to bury that angry part deep within my subconscious. And I know how terrifying it was when that anger re-emerged as hallucinations.

Perhaps the cause of BPD is better explained by a history of childhood abuse, common to so many people with the disorder. One study determined as many as 91 per cent of people with the disorder reported experiencing some form of childhood abuse. Ninety-two per cent were neglected. Those with the disorder are over thirteen times more likely to report childhood adversity or trauma than those without mental illness. When compared to clinical controls, people with BPD experienced abuse at a higher rate than those with mood disorders, psychosis, or other personality disorders. Any type of child abuse can lead to permanent neurological changes in the victim's brain that impair functioning, emotional regulation, impulse control, coping skills, interpersonal skills, and cognitional skills— all symptoms of BPD. The prevalence of abuse histories in people with the disorder might also explain why complex PTSD co-occurs so frequently.

But what constitutes abuse is in the eye of the beholder. Acts I considered abusive weren't necessarily seen that way by others. Violence is relative. It becomes less stark the more a person experiences it. Could I call myself neglected if I rarely went hungry? If I received medical care when I needed it? If I was clean and well dressed? Neglect is relative too.

There's room for people with BPD who don't have abuse histories, just as there are people who were abused who didn't develop the disorder. It's thought that one significant predictor of the disorder is the emotional denial of a child's experiences by their caregiver. This aligns with BPD expert Marsha Linehan's biosocial theory of the disorder, which hypothesizes that BPD emerges in people who were born with biological vulnerabilities and socialized in specific environments. These environments weren't necessarily abusive, but they were invalidating. According to Linehan's manual, "An invalidating environment is one in which communication of private experiences is met by erratic, inappropriate, and extreme responses." An invalidating environment has two characteristics: an intolerance toward the expression of private emotional experiences, and a rejection of emotional displays that communicate to a child that their emotions should be coped with internally without parental support. This results in children who don't learn how to understand, regulate, or tolerate their feelings.

An invalidating environment was easier to reconcile as the cause of my BPD. Invalidation is unintentional. A parent could inadvertently invalidate their child while making their best efforts. Abuse or neglect is a choice (or lack thereof). It requires less emotional pain to accept that I was born into a family that couldn't cater to my unique needs but might have wanted to if they had possessed the necessary tools.

It's also possible I inherited the illness. Genetics are thought to play a role in the development of BPD. A person with a first-degree family member with the disorder is three to four times more likely to have it themselves. A series of studies conducted by researchers at the University of Toronto found that family members of people with BPD have similar brain structures and personality traits. Relatives of people with the disorder showed more personality traits associated with impulsivity and emotional dysregulation, and they were also more likely to be depressed or have a substance use disorder. Family members even reacted to facial expressions in the same manner as their loved ones with BPD. People with the disorder are more sensitive to facial expressions that communicate threats like fear. A 2021 study found their relatives were too. When shown a sad expression, both people with BPD and their relatives took longer to understand the emotion and were more likely to associate it with fright. The behaviours and reactions that define the disorder may be passed on through families.

My therapist was less concerned with how I developed my BPD. Instead, she was focused on unburdening the parts of myself that carried around my difficult childhood memories.

"Have you found her? That young part of you with the house-coat belt around her throat?" my therapist asked.

I let my vision blur. In my mind's eye, I was back in my childhood bedroom with the drunk-tank-pink walls, the pink-and-white striped comforter, and the roses stencilled along the walls' border. Six-year-old me stood in front of the mirror with the housecoat tie draped around her shoulders.

"I found her."

"Great." My therapist's voice filtered into the bedroom like a principal reading the morning announcements over the classroom loudspeaker. "Can you ask her if there's something she wants to tell us? Something she wants us to hear? Something she needs?"

I watched tears form in Little Me's eyes. Big heaving sobs racked her slim shoulders. A wail like a fire alarm escaped her lips. I crouched down so we were eye to eye. She told me she wanted her stepdad to leave. Each word forced out with a sob. She missed her mother—or at least the woman she was before she married.

"Aw, yeah, that makes so much sense," my therapist said. "Can you tell her you understand how she feels? Let her know that you see how brave and capable she's been and how much she's had to take on."

I rubbed Little Me's back. Her shirt was damp with hot sweat. As I spoke, her tears slowed. Her whimpers gave way to deep hiccups that sent shockwaves across her chest.

"Can you ask her if you can remove the tie from her neck?"

Little Me's mouth was still pulled into a deep frown, but she nodded. I took the terrycloth between my thumbs and forefingers. I lifted it from her shoulders, which drooped less in response. Little Me asked if there was something wrong with her. Was her stepdad right about her?

"No," my therapist said. "Everything she's feeling is a normal reaction to her environment. I think we should take her to a place where she can feel safe. But first, let's unburden her from the emotions she's experiencing, so she doesn't have to carry them around anymore."

At my therapist's prompting, I placed two magical boxes at Little Me's feet: one for all the good things she wanted to bring with her and one for all the bad things she wanted to leave behind. The good box shimmered, glowing a clean bright white. Little Me and I filled it with her brown teddy bear, the pale-yellow blanket she liked to smooth against the blade of her index finger when she was upset, her mother drifting in her robe through the quiet dawn, her grandparents and the comforting scent of their laundry detergent. The bad box was the bloody pink of raw meat. Together, we filled it with Little Me's loneliness and confusion, her stepdad's snapping teeth, the interior of his truck, her bladder infections, her swollen lips, her sore body.

"What would you like to do with the bad box?" my therapist asked.

"Burn it," we said.

The flames licked the pink box. Its edges darkened and curled until it collapsed in on itself. Sparks sprayed into the air. Dark plumes of smoke collected into heavy clouds at the ceiling. Standing there in my mind's eye with Little Me, watching all those emotions and memories turn to ash, I felt a lightness spreading across my chest and into my shoulders.

When the fire burned out, I let Little Me dance and laugh in the smoking ashes. Her socks turned black with soot. When she was breathless from jumping and giggling, I hefted the white box onto my hip and took her hand. We walked off to a safer place.

PINK PLASTIC PLAYHOUSE

It happened in the gloomy corner of Uxbridge's premiere watering hole. The town pub. Grizzled regulars spooned the bar. It was late spring but warm enough that the leather banquette stuck to my bare legs like a fly trap. I wore my best denim skirt even though entry only required the presence of a shirt and shoes. At fifteen years old, I was deeply self-conscious and incredibly vain. I had wanted to look my best for the rare surprise outing.

My mother, an aunt I'll call Lena, and I were seated away from the other patrons, back near the dartboards and bathrooms. The table's surface was littered with papers. Copies of emails I had exchanged with my biological father, who I had never met.

He left before I was born because he wasn't ready to be a parent. My mother had shown me a legal agreement she told me that my biological father had signed forfeiting custody in exchange for not paying child support to prove he never wanted me.

Tears flooded my eyes, but I wouldn't let them fall. I didn't want it to get back to any of the kids at high school that I had cried in public. This was a town small enough that my mother would learn from another mom she bumped into at the grocery store that I'd lost my virginity. I wasn't going to give anyone the satisfaction.

My mom held up one of the emails to my biological father and asked why I had written that my stepdad had hurt me.

"Because I wanted my real dad to know what he left me with."

"But it's not true," my mom said. She crossed her arms tight against her chest.

"What do you mean?" Aunt Lena asked me. Her job involved working with troubled youth. She had clearly been brought in to play mediator.

I rolled my eyes. This was the last place I wanted to discuss something so private. I leaned across the table, speaking quietly, my words travelling through clenched teeth. "He hit me, threw me across the room, pushed me down the stairs. I told Grandma Kath and Grampa Joe about it when I was, like, six? Remember?"

Grandma Kath and Grampa Joe were my stepdad's parents. They had raised a terrifying son, but I had always felt safe with them. After I told them what was happening, the physical aggression stopped.

"They never mentioned anything to me." My mom looked at her sister and shook her head like she was trying to knock the thought from her brain.

"You knew!" I whined. "You had to."

"What's clear is things aren't going very well in your family right now," Aunt Lena said. She asked if I would get counselling to improve my relationship with my stepdad. I declined. Like a roll of film, there would be no salvaging the relationship after the family secrets were exposed. I wished I had never found my biological father through an Internet search. I had hoped he might save me from my fragile family circumstances, but my contact with him had only made the dynamic more tenuous.

"Maybe it would be best if you moved in with your Aunt Elaine," my mom said. My aunt Elaine lived in Richmond Hill, a town forty-five minutes away. She had a husband and twin daughters under the age of two.

The tears I had been holding back slipped down my cheeks in hot streams.

"You can finish up grade ten here," my mother said. She began to cry too. "Sometimes, mothers and daughters aren't meant to live together. They have a better relationship if they live apart. I moved out when I was your age."

"Why do I have to be the one to leave?" I asked why my stepdad couldn't move.

"It's not that simple," my mom said. She dabbed her cheeks with Kleenex from her purse. "I have your brother to think of."

I winced. My twelve-year-old younger brother, my mother's child with my stepdad. In photos of us as children, I smiled or sulked, but he never looked at the camera. He was always looking up at me.

"Okay," I said. "I'll move."

Being asked to leave home was upsetting. But it wasn't surprising. In the days after the decision was made, I realized part of me had always been waiting for the moment I'd be left to fend for myself. Maybe it was because abandoned children, orphans, and runaways were pivotal characters in the literature I'd consumed. I couldn't pick up a children's or young adult book without finding one—*Emily of New Moon*, *The Secret Garden*, *Heidi*, *Oliver Twist*, *A Series of Unfortunate Events*, the wizarding series that must not be named. But maybe I was simply drawn to books where children were left alone. Perhaps there was a buried scrap of my intuition that knew I'd need the lessons I could learn from those stories.

Like our pudgy grey-and-white childhood cat, Mindy, who peed all over the laundry once my stepdad and his German shepherd moved in, I was sent away to a relative's house. For good.

✳

About a year later, my uncle and I took a drive in his boxy silver Cadillac, which smelled like cigarette smoke and stale fast-food grease. We stopped near the movie theatre in Richmond Hill where I worked part-time. The car windows were wrapped in darkness made more oppressive by a heavy tint. The atmosphere in the car was dense and uncomfortable. I kept my gaze fixed on my jeans.

"Your aunt Elaine tells me you want to move out," my uncle said.

I nodded and began to stutter an explanation and an apology. Living at my aunt and uncle's house was so different from home. They had only ever parented infants, and it showed. My weekday curfew was six p.m. I had to sign a contract stipulating the terms of my behaviour after I was caught underage drinking when I called an ambulance for a friend with alcohol poisoning. When I skipped class, something my parents allowed so long as I kept my grades up, my uncle grounded me. He chastised me for eating too much of their food. Back home, anything in the fridge or cupboards had been fair game.

My anxiety sharpened painfully in Richmond Hill. One night, I had swallowed half a bottle of Tylenol. I woke up the next morning unable to speak coherently and promptly fainted onto the tiled kitchen floor. I explained the incident as a flu bug. Maybe if I had been honest with my aunt and uncle, it wouldn't have come to this. But honesty didn't come easy in adolescence.

My uncle cut me off before I could try to make him understand. "You're sixteen so no one can stop you if you want to go," he said. His voice was a raspy growl. "But I think it's a really stupid idea." I nodded again.

"If you leave, there's no coming back. I've spoken to your grandparents, your mother, your aunts—we're all finished with you if you move out."

I wasn't sure how my relationship with my uncle had become so adversarial. We had been close when I was a preteen and started to discover Nirvana and contemporary pop-rock, much to his pleasure. I had gone to the real estate magazine office where my uncle worked on Take Your Daughter to Work Day in grade nine since my stepdad didn't really have a job to take me to.

"We won't want to hear from you, so there'll be no running to us if you need money or realize you've made a mistake," he said.

I didn't know it then, but my uncle had likely filtered the conversations he had with my family about me through a lens of tough love. Some family members claimed he hadn't spoken to them at all. Others insisted they had still wanted to hear from me despite my choices. Regardless, that sentence opened up a wound between me and my uncle that would never properly heal.

"I understand," I said. His speech had convinced me, in the twisted logic of a teenager's mind, that I was better off on my own. I ignored the sense that the sheen of innocence I left Uxbridge with was greying.

"Your decision is final," my uncle said.

"I'll be gone by Mother's Day." And I was.

Data suggests that approximately 20 per cent of unhoused people have BPD. A 2003 article by the U.S.-based National Health Care for the Homeless Council notes that people with BPD are vulnerable to houselessness for the same reasons other people with mental illness are at risk: job loss, lack of family support, or substance use disorder. "But their tendency to have volatile relationships with everyone around them—including spouses, bosses, coworkers, landlords, and clinicians—and their inability to trust others make it especially difficult for them to maintain economic and residential stability."

The few months I lived in my friend Olivia's household, just one block over from my aunt and uncle's home, held the most blissful moments of peace I'd find in my adolescence. She was the first friend I had who openly lived with a mental illness. By fifteen, I had recognized that I was depressed, anxious, and struggling with an eating disorder, but when I had tried to talk to my friends from Uxbridge about it, I was often met with scorn or judgment. I didn't have to hide my struggles from Olivia. I could be vulnerable.

On weekday mornings, I dressed and did my makeup in a spare room that had belonged to Olivia's older sister before she moved out. Once I was ready, I slipped into Liv's dim bedroom, crawled beneath her white duvet, and snuggled up close to her.

"Liv?" I asked. I brushed strands of her bleach-blonde hair away from her pale neck. "You coming to school today?"

She grunted and hugged the blankets into her chest. "I'm too depressed. Will you tickle my neck?"

My fingertips danced lightly across her soft skin. Liv sighed. Beyond the door, her mother yelled that she was going to miss the bus if she didn't get up. Spooning beneath the fairy lights strung around Liv's window, all the uncertainty I experienced about striking out on my own faded away. I felt safe.

It turned out Richmond Hill suited me a little better than Uxbridge. My new high school had advanced placement courses, which were far more engaging than anything my old school offered. The town was bigger and more anonymous, and in that anonymity, I found liberation. I found my voice with a new boisterous friend group who weren't afraid to raise eyebrows, celebrated my eccentricities, and encouraged me to step outside my comfort zone in a way I never felt I could in gossipy Uxbridge with its pervasive Christian values. I laughed louder. I began to put words to feelings I had never vocalized. I did things I had only seen in the movies. I had celebrated my sweet sixteen at a rave with Olivia and another girlfriend, and we had convinced some guys we found wandering the street at five a.m. during Toronto's annual Nuit Blanche art festival to take us back to their dorm room to crash. I was free to be whatever I wanted. My past was behind me. There was only the present.

But the pendulum would soon swing back. A teenager makes a poor tenant. The summer sun faded and it was time for me to leave

Olivia's. I lasted a month renting a room in an apartment on Major Mackenzie Drive. On my seventeenth birthday, I was asked to leave. I was about to place a 130-pound strain on my friends' shoulders with my constant need for shelter. A weight they were too young to bear. I would have to be small again to survive.

✳

The sky looked like the ripe skin of a peach. The sunrise air blew goosebumps across my flesh. My shoes raked against the sidewalk. Shaded windows slept on both sides of the block, oblivious to my footsteps.

I stifled a yawn. It was mild enough to rove until the sun woke, neon signs blinked on, and the silent streets filled with their daily scuttle. But the joint I had smoked an hour ago begged me to snooze a bit before the world rose.

I slipped into a narrow passage between detached houses. I listened for human movement from within the walls, but there was only an early bird's solitary song. The gate latch opened with a generous whisper.

Beyond the cobblestone patio, a pink plastic playhouse sat in the grass. It was sized for my aunt's twins but boasted a delicious square of privacy behind a wee Dutch door. Even the purple shutters above the replica sink where the girls cooked pretend meals pulled closed.

The plastic door caught on a scruff of turf, but I heaved it open with my shoulder. A quick crawl in revealed the lawn floor was already sprinkled with morning dew. I rooted around a deck box and found a deflated kiddie pool to spread on the ground. I crept back into my plastic home, fluffed my purse into a pillow, and fell asleep to cricket chirps.

✳

Abraham Maslow's hierarchy of needs proposes that human actions are motivated by certain physical and psychological necessities. The needs considered vital to survival are physiological: food, shelter, water, clothing, and sleep.

The practicalities of meeting these needs while I was housing insecure required some adjustment and resourcefulness. I had no car, nor could I afford one, so I lived primarily out of a series of oversized purses that held everything from toiletries to clean underwear to drugs to homework assignments. My purse's depth was as infinite as a magician's hat.

My high school locker functioned like a storage unit. It's where I kept coursework, changes of clothes, dirty laundry, spare boots and shoes, socks, notebooks filled with angsty teen poetry, a shelf's worth of books, spare phone chargers, and a toothbrush and toothpaste. I also had a small locker with no lock at the movie theatre where I worked. There, I kept my uniform, work shoes, and a hairbrush.

The rest of my possessions were blown about like dandelion seeds on the wind. My grandparents had stored my plastic drawers, snow globes, and childhood trinkets. I kept extra clothes at my aunt and uncle's house even after I moved out and, eventually, at my grandmother's. I borrowed friends' clothes with abandon, leaving my own at their places. I swapped their clothes out with other friends'. Unexpected dresses and sweaters popped up in closets behind me like weeds.

Eating on the road required creativity but was certainly possible. Eating healthy was not. My diet that year consisted of movie theatre popcorn, Tim Hortons bagels, free pizza from Pizza Pizza (a friend worked there), Domino's cinnamon sticks (a splurge), tangerines from Metro the morning after raves, fries or cookies from the high school cafeteria, McDonald's Happy Meals with apple slices and milkshakes, combos from the mall's Manchu Wok, bags of trail mix and candy from Bulk Barn.

Whenever I could, I ate at friends' houses. There was grilled cheese made using multiple kinds of cheese and a garlic spread by a friend's Italian father that I'll never replicate or forget. A seemingly unending supply of baked goods, full chocolate bars, and Pop-Tarts filled the cupboards of a different home. We ordered in Chinese food or pizza to the houses of latchkey kids left to fend for themselves.

Maintaining my hygiene was also challenging. During my time on the road, I was always a bit grubby. I showered at friends' houses when I could, gave myself whore's baths in the staff washroom at my part-time job, and flipped my underwear inside out to get another day out of them. I used the local gym's showers and hot tub whenever I could take advantage of a friend's guest pass. I brushed face powder in my hair to minimize the grease and rarely washed off my makeup. I plucked my eyebrows in the high school bathroom.

Being the only person in my friend group living rough had its benefits. When we got high and wandered through subdivisions under construction, busting into whatever half-finished house caught our fancy, we pretended how we'd decorate the rooms and who would live where. I was always bequeathed the biggest bedroom in our imaginary games.

✳

"When ur roommate leavin?" I texted a guy in my roster. My Motorola Razr and the numbers within functioned like a sailor's SOS. Instead of Morse code, I used T9. I needed to find a safe place for the night if I didn't want to cry myself to sleep in an empty playground with only the low-slung moon watching out for me. That night, I searched for a lifebuoy from a twenty-something movie theatre employee who lived in a cramped basement apartment near my high school.

My phone vibrated. "I think were hoping 4 a 3some??" the message read.

I rolled my eyes in the bus shelter and winced as I shifted my purse from one aching shoulder to the next.

"Not going 2 happen," I typed. "No spit roasts. Only group sex w other girls."

"Fine," he messaged back. "Come over anyway."

An hour later, my palms were pressed into the biting brick exterior of the movie theatre employee's rental. My pants were pushed to my ankles. Menstrual blood tickled my thighs. I angled my hips so it dripped onto dead grass. The movie theatre employee's staccato breaths echoed off the darkened houses we were rammed between.

I closed my eyes to hone in on the pleasure, and for a moment, that's all there was. Pleasure. Rapture. The only sensation within a body that was anesthetized to living nowhere in particular. The movie theatre employee convulsed into me.

"You good?" I asked. I glanced over my right shoulder.

He zipped up his pants over tree-trunk thighs and nodded. He wasn't much of a talker.

"Cool." I pulled up mine. "I'm super tired. I'm going to crash."

I cleaned up in the narrow basement bathroom using a mouldy towel over a rusting porcelain sink flecked with beard hairs. I crawled into the movie theatre employee's double bed in the middle of his studio apartment. I fell into his expansive cotton duvet the way a dehydrated person might fall into a pool of fresh water after being lost at sea. Every cell in my body soaked up the comfort the mattress brought. His pony-tailed roommate pouted from the pullout couch.

In a dissertation about what people with BPD experience when they're abandoned or rejected by family members whom they rely on for care, Laurie O'Boyle wrote, "[It] involves unbearable pain for an extended time during and after the event. [The person with BPD] finds ways to numb herself to avoid feeling. Altering her bodily experience allows her to manage and transform her pain—in a healthy direction if she is athletic, or through other ways of coping such as dissociating, self-cutting, substance abuse, or sexual promiscuity."

Promiscuity in people with BPD could stem from a fear of abandonment—one of the disorder's primary symptoms. One study found that inpatient adolescent girls with BPD had a significantly lower ability to refuse sex than other inpatient teen-agers who engaged in risky sexual behaviour. This trend doesn't end in adolescence. Research conducted on adults with BPD found the fear of abandonment is significantly correlated with sexual compliance and a person's willingness to engage in or be coerced into unwanted sex.

But casual sex can serve as more than a self-destructive coping mechanism for women and girls who fall at the intersection of BPD and houselessness. It's a survival strategy. Unhoused and runaway populations have the highest odds of engaging in survival sex, which is the exchange of sex for money, shelter, or other necessities of life. Nearly half of women with BPD who have engaged in survival sex reported experiencing high levels of abandonment in their lifetime.

Risky behaviour, including unsafe sex, is common for people with BPD. We struggle with impulse control, which can present in habits like reckless spending, substance use disorders, or impulsive sexual behaviour. People with BPD are more likely to engage in casual sexual relationships, start having sex earlier, report a greater number of partners, and appear to be more preoccupied with sex in general.

Casual sex has real health risks: unwanted pregnancy, sexually transmitted infections, and higher odds of a cancer diagnosis. However, attitudes that pathologize a woman's sexuality also cause harm. One study demonstrated that women who were perceived as more open to casual sex were seen as less able to make their own decisions and attributed a limited moral status. Among prominent anti-promiscuous attitudes is the stereotype that women who have sex with multiple partners have low self-esteem; however, recent research found no significant correlation between a woman's sexual behaviour and her self-worth.

Instead, women with BPD were more likely to experience low self-esteem and poor psychological well-being when their trauma responses, including promiscuity, were framed as medically or psychologically abnormal.

In the article "Women at the Margins," authors Clare Shaw and Gillian Proctor write that "BPD is the latest manifestation of historical attempts to explain away the strategies which some women use to survive and resist oppression and abuse, by describing these strategies as symptomatic of a disturbed personality [or] pathology."

The line between a mental illness and a reasonable reaction can get blurry when compounded by housing insecurity. Imagine you're an unhoused seventeen-year-old girl. Your feet are blistered raw, and cold penetrates your bones. You've lost track of the steps, the hours, and the hope you started your trek with. There's no pillow to rest your head upon at the end of this road, no hamper in which to deposit the dirty underwear zipped into the purse that chews on your shoulder, no warm meal to sate the void in your belly. There are only shuffling steps in a protracted night.

You have two choices. You can keep plodding along until red streaks bleed across the sky like the horizon cut itself open to show off its heart. Your stomach will stay as empty as your wallet. You'll trip on an uneven sidewalk and flay your numb fingers. You'll bide time until a Tim Hortons opens and you can rinse out your wounds and rest your head on a table blotched with bagel crumbs.

Or you can answer the text from the drug dealer you infrequently hook up with. His blaring voice makes you nauseous, but he'll dispatch his driver to collect you in a decaying Civic. The heated car will melt your frozen hands and nourish your tender muscles. You'll have to allow the dealer's wormy lips to make a feast of your flesh, but there will be a bed to sleep in and a refrigerator to scavenge.

If you choose the latter, do you consider it a logical reaction to the circumstances described? Or an indicator of a disordered personality?

Twice a month, I rode the lumbering blue Viva bus north to Aurora. These trips were often without cost. The Viva, or "Free-va" as my adolescent associates and I called it, basically operated on the honour system. And we were a long way from honourable. Richmond Hill's unvaried clusters of townhouses gave way to sweeping grounds encircling towering estates. The warbled speaker called my stop in the historic downtown, a quaint street dotted with Victorian and Italianate shops. The bus grunted to the ground. Beyond the charming brick facades, through a teeming plaza, was a nondescript office building. Kinark Child and Family Services.

My counsellor and I met in a stale conference room washed pale by buzzing fluorescent lights. The walls muffled the wails of children and sighs of teenagers in the waiting room. There was no supple couch to recline on like I had seen in the movies. We sat diner-style, a scarred surface of particleboard between us.

According to the psychologist who joined our sessions once a month to adjust my new antidepressants, I was suffering from major depressive disorder and generalized anxiety disorder. (BPD is frequently misdiagnosed.) But therapy hadn't been a possibility until I left home. It violated the rules my stepdad chipped and chiselled into me over twelve long years until he had left his thumbprints all over my brain. Therapy contradicted his rule that whatever happened within our walls stayed there, that I wasn't to run my mouth off to people with sob stories about how hard I had it. I had to be careful about what I said in public. Anything could be used against the family. My counsellor respected my concerns in this regard, including my forceful protests against involving the Children's Aid Society.

"How are you feeling?" Sandra asked. Her dimples popped to sandwich her cherubic smile. Sandra was a hug in human form. She radiated comfort, which filled the space with needed warmth.

"Anxious. And sad. My mom and I met up for lunch. I sort of word-vomited a bunch of feelings onto her." After a strained interlude, my relationship with my mother existed solely within restaurant walls during the odd lunch break. These reunions were often lachrymose and seemed to add weight to my bones.

"How did that go?" Sandra asked.

"I waited until the drive back to school—you know my aversion to public vulnerability—and told her how alone and isolated I feel. It seems like there's no one to catch me if I fall. I thought her love was supposed to be unconditional. Instead, it's like she's given up on me."

"And how did she react?" Sandra's job, I realized, was primarily about listening to me. It felt good to be heard.

"She told me that she loved me, but had to go back to work. She was crying a bit. She sent a nice email that afternoon. It said she would always be in my corner even when we didn't get along. And that she'd like to see me more often. It was really great—until the end."

Sandra nodded me along. The key card that hung from a lanyard around her neck clanked against the table's edge.

I attempted to contort my voice into my mother's, but her voice was mine. Mimicking it created a cartoon: "'I already lived through what you have but much worse.' She reminded me she was on her own at my age but didn't have any family support. I guess she only talked to her parents once or twice during her time on the road."

"It sounds like your mom is trying to empathize," Sandra said. "Just in her own way."

"I know. And I feel guilty that I'm frustrated. I get that she's trying to connect and be loving, but I'd like to be allowed to have my own experience without it being compared to someone else's. You know?"

Sandra nodded. "Could you say that to your mom?"

"No. I don't want to risk losing her support. I don't want her to dislike me." I pushed back from the table. "It's just all too much. There are so many feelings swirling around in my head, and anytime I pause to feel them I want to shut down."

"Sometimes, having a better understanding of our emotions can help us feel less overwhelmed," Sandra said. She pulled out a few cognitive behavioural therapy handouts about the three component model of emotions and slid them over to me. The file of skills she brought to our sessions was the part of therapy that made the most sense. It was like homework—the only area of my life I had no trouble with.

We filled out the worksheets together. We drew arrows between words like *frustration*, *guilt*, and *avoidance* until they formed a spiral of distress. The face of Sandra's wristwatch told me our session was almost at its end.

"Is there anything else you'd like to talk about today?"

There was—the part of my life that was inescapable, the nonstop search for shelter that had created a knot in my belly that wouldn't untangle. "No," I lied.

I minimized the impact certain parts of my life had on me when I was with Sandra. The parts that might splinter what was left of my family home. I tiptoed around slivers of truth because honesty was what had led me to this precarious reality. Sandra's sympathy was welcome though. With time, I wanted her to admire me. I wanted her to feel like her efforts were making a difference. So, I chipped and chiselled myself into a shape I thought she might like.

The province found me after I panicked during drama class. My berserk breath and hysterical bulging eyes alerted a friend, who told the teacher, who sent me to the vice-principal's office, who spoke with my guidance counsellor, who called a social worker in a miserable game of Broken Telephone.

Months elapsed before the social worker pulled up to my high school in a corroded van and drove me to a group home in Markham, just off Highway 7. The house was unassuming. It looked like all the others on the block. A juvenile tree ripe with tight green buds leaned from the force of the wind at the lawn's edge.

"Do I have to stay here?" Blood pulsed through my ears as I sat in the passenger seat.

"Only if you want to," the social worker said. "The school called us to explore your options, but you're over sixteen. You can do whatever you want."

Inside, I toured a middle-class home cut up into a half-dozen bedrooms. Chore lists and house rules were tacked to the walls. The room that could become mine showed marks of being lived in by many before. In the kitchen, a guy who looked to be about my age ate from a bag of chips labelled with his name. He told me living there was okay, he guessed.

"So, what do you think?" the social worker asked on the way back to her van. "Should I let the support worker know you'll take the free room?"

"I saw that the curfew is eleven. My job at the movie theatre sometimes doesn't let out until one in the morning." I pulled a seat-belt pocked with burn holes across my chest.

"Then you'd have to quit," she said.

The group home shrank in the side-view mirror. "I'm not sure what to do."

"It sounds like you already have a pretty good system worked out on your own. And there's a girl right below you on the waiting list who's fleeing from an abusive environment. She could really use the room."

The social worker was right. My life on the road had taken on a familiar rhythm. One night, shivering on a park bench, my fingertips throbbing, I flipped my phone open and closed. The battery life withered away. I shrieked into the dark cloak of a woodland behind a local Catholic school. I summoned my aunt Elaine's number on the phone's screen, took a frosty breath, and told her I made a mistake. Following intense bargaining, my aunt and uncle had agreed to let me stay in their spare room twice a week on nights that I worked.

A month or two later, a cousin had vacated a room in my grandparents' wartime bungalow in Scarborough. The two-hour transit trip wasn't possible on the nights I worked late. With only two months until graduation, I didn't want to switch schools again. But it was a safe landing whenever I couldn't find a place to sleep closer to my high school. In the mornings, Grandma Kath toasted a bagel with cheese to include in the lunch she packed for me. Once in a while, my grampa Joe, a surly Sicilian with a greying ducktail hairdo, drove me all the way to Richmond Hill. Before he retired, he was a long-haul trucker. He knew a thing or two about what an endless stretch of lonely road could do to a person.

I turned back to the social worker. "Give the room to her then," I said.

The social worker dropped me off at high school, wished me luck, and that was the last I ever saw of her.

✳

In the 1999 book *The Impact of Multiple Childhood Trauma on Homeless Runaway Adolescents*, author Michael DiPaolo wrote that predictors of BPD in unhoused and runaway youth included psychological abuse or neglect and unsupportive communities. Drawing on Theodore Millon's research, DiPaolo notes that children raised in environments where there's emotional neglect "must rely on their community to provide the backup to compensate and repair the family system defects and failures." When a community fails to provide these resources, unhoused adolescents don't learn how to manage their impulses. They become, as Millon noted, "victims of their own growth."

If I had a more supportive community during my time couch-surfing—and I'm not referring to my peers but to the adults whom I occasionally collided with—would I have avoided BPD? Or was it already too late for me?

My guidance counsellor was a broomstick of a man. His eyes grew overly bright when he was tasked with assisting a student in an actual crisis instead of merely doling out university brochures to confused kids trying to decide where to spend their parents' money.

He had stopped me in the hallway on my way from the smokers' pit to check in about my university acceptance letters. Guelph and Laurentian would take me in, but Ryerson University (as it was known then) was still considering me. It was the only institution I wanted to call home. It had the best journalism program in the country.

"Well, let's just see what we can do about that," the guidance counsellor said. He had led me through a snarl of students on their way to class, lunch, or to smoke weed in the forested parkland that clung to the school's periphery.

In his office, he cradled the phone between his shoulder and ear and held up a single finger. My eyes drifted to the pile of pamphlets about post-traumatic stress disorder, methamphetamines, and sexually transmitted diseases scattered about his desk.

"Admissions, please," he said into the line.

"Ah, hello, yes." The guidance counsellor sat up straighter in his office chair. He introduced himself and explained where he was calling from. "I'd like to inquire about an applicant to your journalism program—Miranda Newman. Yes, wait-listed. That's her."

He shifted the phone from his left ear to his right. "I'm sitting with her in my office right now, and she's quite upset."

My cheeks filled with blood. I was far from upset. Sleeping rough had shown me layers of grief I had never imagined existed.

"I'm hoping I might be able to sway your admission decision. Miranda is one of the most exceptional students I've had the pleasure of guiding. She would make a wonderful addition to your student body, but she comes from unusual circumstances." The guidance counsellor paused to smooth a crease that had formed between his brow with his index and middle figure.

"Well, yes. You see, she doesn't really live anywhere. Homeless, yes, I suppose that's right. But through it all, still able to maintain quite a high average in primarily gifted courses, which I'm sure you'll agree is impressive." The guidance counsellor gave me a thumbs-up.

"Why didn't she mention it in her application? Oh well, she's pretty independent and not always the best at asking for help—not that I can blame her. Oh, really?" The guidance counsellor's smile spread across his face like a sunrise reaching over a shadowed land. "Thank you. That's fantastic news. I'll tell her right away." The receiver embraced the phone with a gentle click. "You're in. You're going to Ryerson."

＊

By the last week of August, when autumn was already whispering in the evening air, I signed a lease for shared student accommodation in downtown Toronto. The student loan program was generous to people like me who applied under the "broken family" category, which meant they only took my movie theatre income into consideration when determining how much money to distribute. Loans and help from both sets of grandparents turned the dreams of a roof over my head into a real stucco ceiling. Since graduation, my family's demeanour toward me had, for the most part, thawed. They were able to imagine big things for me again.

Grandma Kath and Grampa Joe came with me to get the keys and lay claim to my preferred bedroom by marking it with the few boxes of my possessions that survived the year.

"Oh, I just love this place," Grandma Kath said. We were looking out my new window on the sixth floor onto Gerrard Street below. A firetruck screamed past pedestrians who hurried along the sidewalk. "I think you're going to be very happy here."

"Not too shabby, Doo Dah." Grampa Joe said. "Where do you want this rug?"

Among the possessions we hauled from Scarborough was a prized sheepskin rug given to me by my mother's parents.

"Unroll it. I'm going to sleep on it here tonight."

"Without a bed?" Grandma Kath's eyes turned into full moons behind her glasses. "Why don't you just come back to our place tonight? You'll be more comfortable there."

"Nope. I want to sleep here."

"If she wants to sleep on the floor, let her, Kath." Grampa Joe spread the rug onto the black-and-white tiles.

I had a place to live again. But I was lucky. Some unhoused people with BPD never find their way home.

THE DIFFICULT PATIENT

"The most notorious is the diagnosis of borderline personality disorder. This term is frequently used within the mental health professions as little more than a sophisticated insult. As one psychiatrist candidly confesses, 'As a resident, I recalled asking my supervisor how to treat patients with borderline personality disorder, and he answered, sardonically, 'You refer them.'"

—JUDITH LEWIS HERMAN, *Trauma and Recovery*

"I don't belong here!" My yell clawed up the emergency room walls.

A harried nurse shoved a tiny paper cup at me with a small pill inside. She told me to take it. That the pill would help.

"Let me out of here," I screamed. "I don't want your pills."

"I'm trying to be patient with you," the nurse said. "But I'll strap you down if I have to."

The psych ward is where the world drops dead. It's the place I was trapped between beginnings and endings. I arrived between the end of my third semester of university and the beginning of my final year; at the end of my first serious relationship, the end of my pregnancy, the end of my bedbug-infested rental in St. James Town in

77

Toronto; and at the beginning of hallucinations—red iridescent orbs that obscured my field of vision and indecipherable whispers; at the beginning of a lust for self-destruction so powerful that every blunt object offered a way out.

Inside the hospital, I couldn't feel the heat wave that was plaguing Toronto and had killed at least ten people in Montreal. I couldn't find out if I'd been approved for a new apartment on Broadview Avenue, just up the street from Jack Layton's campaign office. I couldn't attend the first SlutWalk, organized after Toronto police constable Michael Sanguinetti suggested "women should avoid dressing like sluts" if they didn't want to be assaulted. All I could do was watch the nurse's angry eyes watch me. She waited for the Ativan beneath my tongue to dissolve. And waited for me to stop being such a difficult patient.

I didn't know it yet—I wouldn't be formally diagnosed with BPD for another seven years—but certain undertones of my behaviour put me in direct opposition with the people responsible for helping me. According to a 2002 study assessing mental health workers' attitudes toward people with BPD, "Over 80 per cent of staff viewed this population as difficult to work with, and indeed, more difficult to treat than [people] with other mental illnesses." A 2021 protocol paper determined that institutional stigma especially affected people with BPD in crisis who presented to emergency departments.

✳

Everything was white in the locked unit of the suburban hospital's psychiatric intensive care ward. White tiles pooled the reflection from overhead lights like ghostly moons. White walls stood scarred but sturdy. (Primarily) white people floated through the common area in pale robes. White sheets covered beds bolted to the floors. The whiteness filled my mouth like snow. I didn't speak until I saw a colour.

"May I borrow one of those?" I pointed to a box of Crayola crayons by the sharp elbow of a timid woman who sat alone in the common room.

She flinched but gestured to the box. "Go ahead. Anyone can use them," she said. "They're not mine." She pulled a hospital blanket around her bony frame and asked if I'd like to sit with her. A scowling blonde with a scarred red face exited her room and came toward us before I could decide.

"Why are you here?" the angry blonde asked me. She pulled out a chair next to the small woman.

My shocked mouth fell open to answer.

"You don't have to tell her that," the mousy woman said. She pinched the blonde, who stormed back to her room and shouted that I didn't belong in the hospital. The door banged shut behind her and muffled her rage.

The small woman told me not to worry. The angry blonde was just grumpy in the morning.

I had no idea it was morning.

The blonde may not have thought I belonged there, but the admitting psychiatrist sure did. He signed my Form 1, a legal document that committed me to the care of the hospital for seventy-two hours. His white coat had wafted behind him when he breezed into the ER triage room. He had judged me with smug owlish eyes behind his glasses and clipboard. A twist of white hair had fallen across his forehead. I had demanded to be released. I reminded him that I had admitted voluntarily.

"Why should I trust you?" he had asked. "You came to us for help. You were here only an hour before you hyperventilated and asked to be discharged. You're too impulsive to be released. You've failed to convince me otherwise."

In hindsight, I suspect the admitting psychiatrist recognized the symptoms of my BPD, which is why he found me so exasperating. "Some clinicians have described [people] with BPD as manipulative—that is, clinicians believe people with BPD have more control of their emotions and behaviours than consumers with other mental illnesses; and they misbehave—rather than their behaviour being an expression of mental illness," the 2021 protocol paper noted.

Noah moved his hand farther up the page he was colouring. The handcuff that chained him to the chair yanked him back like he was a mad dog lunging on the leash. Noah sighed quietly and hung his substantial head. "I'm not dangerous, you know," he said.

"You don't seem like it." I nodded to the underwater scene Noah was working on. Only a few patches of white remained. "You're pretty good at colouring."

His broad face split into a grin. "I do it a lot with my daughter."

Noah and I sat at a table and coloured like schoolchildren with the angry blonde and the small woman, Connie. Connie had been hospitalized before. In fact, a prior hospitalization was how she met the angry blonde. She told us that the more time we spent outside our room socializing, the more likely the nurses and doctors would think we were getting better. Improvement equalled freedom. Freedom meant a world in motion.

"How old is your daughter?" I asked Noah.

"Three. She's an angel. I'm so worried I won't be able to see her again." Noah capped his marker. "It was just a misunderstanding."

A thumping noise interrupted our conversation. It came from the closed door of a patient's room. I'd heard it on and off since I arrived. There was a fleshy slapping tone to the beating. I asked the others in a whisper if they heard it too.

"It's Nathan hitting himself," the angry blonde said. She yawned widely, revealing black gaps in her mouth. Missing teeth.

I was relieved because I thought I was hallucinating the sounds, but Connie looked concerned. She left the table to get a nurse. The nurse, Connie, and two security guards entered Nathan's room.

A grating scream broke apart the murmurs in the common area. Connie scurried back to the table.

"Everything okay?" I asked. I wasn't sure if I was asking Connie or myself.

"They're giving him a shot," Connie said. "I'm not sure I did the right thing."

The common area was rowdier than usual. It was occupied by out-siders. Families smiled in their summer plumage as colourful as the birds I wished I could hear beyond my hospital window. The pale ghosts that called the ward home gamely nodded or blinked along to conversations. I sat with my granny and my mother and tried to part the chemical clouds that obscured my mind.

My mom asked when I was going to be moved to the open side of the ward. I was only in the locked unit because there weren't any free beds on the other side. Her cheeks were gaunt, and her eyes were rimmed with dark circles.

"I haven't heard." I tried to shrug, but the air felt as heavy as sand. "How long have I been here?"

My granny and my mother looked startled. They were still living with time that was linear and not a puddle of hours to wade in. "Three days," Granny said.

A weak chuckle bubbled through my lips. "That's it?"

Granny decided we were getting to the bottom of the matter. She popped a Tic Tac into her mouth and shook the container at my mother who accepted a mint. I refused. I was at my limit of ingesting pill-shaped things.

"Excuse me." Granny beckoned a nurse in wrinkled turquoise scrubs. "We were told my granddaughter was only meant to be on this side of the ward until a bed becomes free on the open side. It's been three days, and she's getting worse the longer she waits. When is she being moved?"

The nurse looked at me as if I was a piece of gum she'd stepped in. "I have no notes on her being transferred to open."

"You need to check again." Granny used her sternest tone. "Right away."

"I think I would remember something like that." The nurse rolled her eyes but retreated into the fishbowl-like office.

"Quite the attitude on her," Granny said.

I wanted to tell her all the nurses were like that, but I was shaking too violently. My mom noticed the sweat shining on my open palms. "Are you okay?" she asked.

"Di-di-did they forget me?" My stutter only surfaced during times of extreme duress. I looked down at the blue flowers tattooed on my quivering wrists. Forget-me-nots. Not quite a perfect rendering of the ones I used to pick with Granny in the ravine behind her house, nor as dainty as the ones engraved inside her and Grampa's wedding rings, but my own small plea to the world. Forget-me-not.

"We're getting it all figured out," Granny said.

The nurse reappeared. "I'm so sorry." Her temperament had shifted from salty to sweet. "You were right. She was supposed to be on open—no one told me. We're just getting a room ready—"

"And how long will that take?" Granny asked.

"A half hour or so." The nurse left.

"See? All sorted." Granny tucked her Tic Tacs back into her purse. "You just have to stay on these people."

I slammed my fist onto the table. People nearby jumped in their seats. The words gurgled up, beyond my control, rapid-fire like a machine gun spraying senselessly in search of a target. "How am I supposed to get better in a place where they forget me? Do you know how fucking difficult it is to vouch for yourself when time stretches like taffy and dreams are the only semblances of reality—"

"That's enough." Granny nodded in the direction of a nurse, who was watching me rave with narrowed eyes. "Behave yourself or they might not move you."

Before I was admitted, I had assumed mental health professionals were on my side. Or, at the very least, that we shared a common goal: my health and well-being. But that's not necessarily true for people with BPD. A 2013 literature review in *Innovations in Clinical Neuroscience* found that mental health professionals socially distanced themselves from people with BPD, were more defensive and less helpful, and expressed less empathy and more anger when dealing with people with the disorder.

Open was noisier. Patients milled about in street clothes. They zipped through halls decorated with inmate artwork and dry-erase activity calendars to chat with each other. The rooms weren't private like in lockdown. I noted through sneaky glances that they were divided by gender. I didn't have a roommate. Two beds had been available on this side of the ward while I was trapped in lockdown.

There was also a dining area that included a nearly complete kitchen. Decaf coffee spat into my Styrofoam cup. "Hey," a plain middle-aged woman called to me. "I think I know you."

I recognized her from the ER. To distract myself from smashing my head against the tiled floor until I was nothing more than a swirl of grey matter, I had watched this woman and her friend chug jumbo sodas and mash greasy fries into their mouths. Animals don't feed when they're vulnerable. Did they have no sense of self-preservation?

"I think I saw you in emerg," I said.

"Ah, that's it. I'm Laurie." Laurie sat at a table with a man whose frizzy grey hair shot out in every direction. He looked like a wizard.

"And I'm Kenneth," the wizard said. His smile revealed a gap between his two front teeth.

Laurie nodded at my coffee. Her sugar was labelled in one of the kitchen cupboards, she said, and I was welcome to it. I told her I didn't need any, still feeling guilty about the scorn I had heaped on her in the ER, but she jumped to her feet to get it anyway.

"Tell me something," Kenneth said. He hit a perfectly timed pause to draw me into his words. "If you and Laurie came in at the same time, how come you're just getting here now?"

"That's a good question," I said. I felt rage race through my body at the injustice.

Laurie returned to the table with a bag of processed sugar. I told them both about how the staff forgot about me in lockdown.

Laurie frowned. "I was sent up here right away, but I self-admitted."

"I did too." I had to steady my hand's rage shakes as it heaped sugar into my cup. I couldn't understand why Laurie had been treated differently than I was. "Do you have privileges?"

"What do you mean?"

"Do you eat meals with real cutlery? Are you allowed to go out-side?" I heard my patience wear thin. My seventy-two-hour hold had elapsed—the hospital had no legal recourse to hold me—but the nurses wouldn't allow a change in my status until I saw a psychiatrist. The one assigned to me was on vacation.

"Yep," Laurie said. "The doctors are trying to work me up to passes so I can spend time with my son. He's barely a year old."

Something in my own womb tightened. A high-pitched whine filled my ears like a mosquito was trapped inside my head. "So, you didn't self-harm when you came in? Did you tell them you were thinking of killing yourself? Did you tell them you had a plan?"

Laurie curled into herself like a pill bug. "I've been really depressed since I gave birth. I got to the point . . . I don't want to leave my son."

"I'm sorry." I knew I had gone too far in my quest for answers. "Thank you for the sugar. I really hope you get to spend time with your son soon."

This prompted an eloquent diatribe from Kenneth about how the right life force or energy can help a person achieve their goals, which explained his tie-dyed T-shirt and general Deadhead vibes. He pushed a clump of hair, dampened by the speech's vigour, from his forehead. He folded his arms against his chest and leaned back in his seat.

Before my budding journalist's instincts could inquire further, a white-haired woman whose face was weathered and wilted but held a faded loveliness wandered up to us. Her name was Ivy, and she was looking for a girl named Gina. "She's supposed to paint my nails."

"I think she's with a nurse," Laurie said.

Ivy's eyes grew wide like a pale morning glory at first light. "She promised."

"She will, Ivy," Laurie said. "Why don't you sit with us while you wait for her to turn up?"

Ivy's chair was pulled out by a man with light clipped hair flecked with grey. His body jerked with tremors so the chair moved in screeches and bursts. Black circles around his brown eyes made them gleam. He was dressed like a sitcom dad from the eighties in corduroys and a wool sweater. His clothing choice might have struck me as odd if we had been outside to feel the summer heat. But we were in a seasonless place.

"How's the withdrawal today, Sheldon?" Kenneth asked the man.

Sheldon tried to manage an answer, but a girl around my age with bright dyed blonde hair set against sharp black streaks bounded up to us.

"Hey! Hi! Hello!" She greeted us each in turn.

"Hi, Gina." Kenneth smiled. Sheldon chuckled in his quivery way.

Gina clasped her hands to her face like Macaulay Culkin in *Home Alone* when she saw Ivy. "I'm supposed to do your nails! I'll get my stuff. Come with me—" She pulled on Ivy's arm but changed her mind and dropped it. "No! Stay right here. I'll bring everything out."

Gina skipped away. Ivy, ignoring her, trailed after.

The nurse led me to what I thought was a supply closet. It turned out to be a windowless meeting room for my appointment with the on-call psychiatrist—the man who had trapped me here. A few carelessly placed office chairs surrounded a large table. The psychiatrist sat with his hands folded primly on a manila folder with my name on it. He gestured to a seat across from him and asked how I was feeling.

"I want to go home."

"That's what we're here to determine." The doctor opened my file. He asked if I'd had any suicidal thoughts since we last spoke.

"I'm feeling much better." I forced any emotion out of my voice. "But I know I'd feel even better if I could leave. My anxiety isn't good in here." The glaring overhead lights made me feel like I was in an interrogation room.

"You didn't answer the question. And I'm seeing a lot of that impulsivity. One minute you tell me you're feeling fine. The next, you tell me you're anxious—"

"You're twisting my words—"

The doctor held up a veined hand to silence me. "The same thing happened to you when you were admitted. One second you wanted to stay, the next you wanted to leave. How am I supposed to trust you?"

Hidden from the doctor's sight, my fingernails tore into my palms beneath the table until the flesh broke and filled my nails with crescent moons of blood. I wanted to flip over the table and crush this asshole beneath it, but a temper tantrum wouldn't get me out of the hospital. I took a deep breath. "I've done everything the hospital has asked me to. I'm feeling much better, and I would like to be discharged."

"I'm not sure I see that here." He flipped through my folder. "The nurses note you haven't been eating much."

"I'm not eating much because I keep telling the hospital I'm a vegetarian and you keep giving me meat," I said.

"There's no need to get upset now." The doctor scratched something into my file. "Tell me again about the incident with your boyfriend and his balcony. Did you try to jump because you truly wanted to kill yourself or simply because you wanted his attention?"

I dug my nails deeper into my bloody palms. "He is my ex-boyfriend, and no. I tried to jump because of the intensity of my emotions. The pain was excruciating. I think the hormones from before my pregnancy was terminated made my feelings more intense than normal."

The doctor's pen made furious notes. "This most recent abortion was your second? Tell me about the first. I take it this ex-boyfriend wasn't the father?"

"My ex is the only person I've ever been pregnant by."

A static silence hung between us. The doctor seemed to sense he'd crossed a line. He dropped his gaze from mine and cleared his throat. "Your Form 1 is up today."

"It was up yesterday."

"Ah." The doctor frowned. "So it was. Would you consider staying at the hospital voluntarily?"

"No," I answered quickly. Maybe too quickly. "Being here isn't helpful for me."

"I don't agree." He slipped a sheet of paper from the folder. "I think it's better to keep you here a little longer to be sure. I'm signing you onto a Form 3, which means you'll be involuntarily admitted for another two weeks."

"It's not fair," I cried. "I came here voluntarily and I'm being treated like a prisoner for trying to get some help. I've been forgotten, overlooked—"

"No one is treating you like a prisoner. I'm making a decision that's in the best interest of your safety." He clicked his pen and gathered his papers.

The most frustrating aspect of my time in inpatient care was the low opinion the on-call psychiatrist held of me. He made up his mind that I was a certain type of person. A difficult person. A 2006 *Psychiatric Services* review found that BPD was mentioned four times more than any other diagnosis when psychiatrists were asked about the characteristics of difficult patients, even though their behaviours were no more disruptive than people with other diagnoses.

The "difficult" behaviour displayed by people with BPD could result in mental health clinicians keeping people with BPD at arm's length, which, according to a 2006 *Harvard Review of Psychiatry* article, "may also unintentionally stimulate these patients to engage in unhealthy behaviours to cope with such threats (e.g., self-harm behaviours, withdrawal from treatment)."

Ivy and I sat in the television lounge and listened to the summer rain tap against the window. Toni was missing.

I had met Toni a few nights ago at dinner. I had carried my tray through a maze of chair legs until I found a free seat at Ivy's table.

"Christ, you're just a baby," Toni had said. She had dark peppery roots that glowered against her brassy yellow hair. "What on earth are you doing here?"

I had lifted the lid on my dinner tray to find a greying piece of chicken. "Same thing that brings most of us here, I expect."

"Tried to kill yourself and blew it?"

I had laughed for the first time since I came to the hospital.

"That's hardly dinner conversation," Ivy had said.

"It's fine." I had waved a hand over broccoli that had been boiled into a fart of itself. "She's mostly right."

"It's hard to kill a human being," Toni had said. "I took hundreds of pills and still woke up the next morning. I felt like such a piece of shit. Can't even get offing myself right."

"Now, now." Ivy had laid a tissue-papery hand on top of Toni's.

Toni had been given her first pass this afternoon, which allowed her outside for fifteen minutes to smoke. The nurses' station began to buzz like a hive of bees that lost its queen when the staff realized she hadn't signed back in. I heard them call the police to report her missing.

"I bet Toni's sitting beneath a tree on top of a two-four right now," Ivy said. She stared out the window at the moody sky.

"What will happen if they find her?" I asked.

"They'd bring her back here. But they won't find her." Ivy folded her hands in her lap. Gina had painted her fingernails a bright cerulean, like the waves none of us would splash in that summer. "She's lived in this town since she was a girl. She knows where to go and has people to stay with."

"Do you know her well?"

"Oh, sure. It's a small town and we run in the same circles. My ex dated her cousin. She's a real scrapper, Toni. Could always keep up with the guys."

The sleepy monotony of the ward was replaced with a wired and frenetic energy as electric as the storm brewing outside. Clusters of people conspired in the kitchen, whispered unseen in bedrooms, and cast longing glances at the ward's locked double doors.

But if Toni had overdosed, I wondered, maybe she was better off here?

"She was drunk when she did it. When the paramedics brought her in, she tried to give it a shot for a few days. She didn't think it was helping though. She wanted to keep drinking."

Ivy leaned back in her seat, closed her eyes, and sighed deeply enough for her sharp ribs to raise the gauzy cloth of her nightgown. "It takes its toll."

I didn't know if it was Toni's absence, alcoholism, or the psych ward that took its toll. I didn't ask.

※

Dinner's crumbs were wiped from the tables. Evening meds were doled out.

Gina, Kenneth, Sheldon, Laurie, and I gathered around a deck of cards at a dining table. I dealt out eight cards to each person.

"This is called Crazy Eight Countdown. It's a card game I used to play up at my cottage on rainy days. It's good because it lasts a long time."

The best way to whittle away the hours was to play cards. Group therapy, music therapy, art therapy, and pet therapy were cancelled for the summer. During the day, Patrick, an Irishman on the ward, and I played War, a game simple enough that Patrick could play through his Parkinson's and tell me of his life immigrating to Canada from a county in Ireland that I had once visited. We made plans to visit Ireland's rolling emerald hills after we were discharged, though we both knew we'd never make the trip.

At night, whoever was daring enough to fight the drowsy effects of the antipsychotic that we were all prescribed played games that were slightly more complex.

I flipped a face card and set the deck between the five of us. I explained that we discarded our hands by matching the suit or number to the face card or by playing a wild card.

A few nods. "Reminds me of Uno," Gina said. Her chin was tucked into her sweater.

"It's a lot like that," I agreed. "Everybody following?"

A chorus of "yes." Chair legs scraped up to the edge of the table. The gameplay was slow at first. Each player focused as best they could while the rules bounced around their medicated brains. The high that came at night when we fought the meds was a sharp, edgy contrast to the pudding-like passage of time during the day.

Gina played first—a three to change suit to diamonds. She smacked her card down on the table and waggled her eyebrows at the group. Kenneth played a two of diamonds, and Laurie had to pick up two cards. After a few rounds, the pace increased and we were able to have conversations unrelated to the game.

"Look," Laurie hissed and nodded at the nurses' station. "The hunky nurse is back."

It was a male nurse I had noticed while I was still in lockdown. His muscles threatened to burst the seams of his scrubs.

Laurie whistled low and slow. "He's really good-looking."

"I wouldn't mind taking that ride," I said. This set off a case of giggles that persisted and built throughout the game.

"You sure you're ready for this?" Sheldon asked. He stacked a two of clubs and a two of spades atop a two of hearts. He narrowed his eyes and grinned a lopsided smile. "Pick up six, Miranda!"

The group whooped and laughed at my poor luck. A few nurses milling behind the glass of their office shot dirty looks in our direction. The fluorescents in the hallway were off. Darkness obscured the hospital grounds beyond the window.

"Oh, yeah?" I slammed down the queen of spades after I collected my cards. "Pick up eleven, bitches!"

More peals of laughter, which felt like a gust of fresh air blowing away the stale scent that pervaded the psych ward. A nurse with black winged eyeliner marched up to our card game.

"You're all supposed to be in bed," she said.

The laughter dwindled into uneasy chuckles. "We're having fun," I said. "Isn't that a good thing?"

"No." The nurse crossed her arms against her chest. "It's too disruptive."

I stopped to listen to the sounds of the ward. Not a creature stirred.

"I'm sorry—laughter is too disruptive? Laughing is bad?" I asked.

"Go to bed," she said. "Or you'll all be getting shots."

My tablemates grumbled and pulled themselves to their feet. They slowly tidied the cards. The nurse headed back toward the office. A flash of anger shook my frame.

"Hey," I yelled across the room to her. "You're a fucking bitch."

According to a 2008 report about nurses' perceptions of people with BPD, "The core theme was: 'Destructive Whirlwind', which

refers to the nurses perceiving these patients as a powerful, dangerous, unrelenting force that leaves a trail of destruction in its wake."
Nurses are reported to have the lowest self-ratings on empathy
toward those with BPD when compared to other mental health professionals. A 2012 study interviewed seventeen psychiatric nurses
about their feelings toward people with the disorder. Eleven per
cent said that "they would avoid providing a [person] with BPD any
level of care or just a minimal level . . . [and] they would avoid any
interaction with people with BPD until it was completely necessary."
When a nurse did have to interact with a person with BPD, they
would wait until the end of the day when they knew there would be
no time to explore their concerns.

I followed my new roommate, Veronica, down a back staircase.

"We've got to make every second count," she explained. "And
the stairs are faster."

It was my first smoking pass. The on-call psychiatrist had
pulled me into a meeting room while I was wandering the halls,
singing to myself.

He had told me I was ready for privileges like metal cutlery and
smoking passes. He had also told me it would be our last session
together. My assigned psychiatrist was returning from summer
vacation.

Veronica and I burst through a set of doors at the side of the
hospital. Veronica ran ahead, across the parking lot and over a narrow strip of grass, to the sidewalk where a group of people were

bunched beneath a hazy cloud of cigarette smoke. I ran behind her with my arms flung to the sky like I was trying to hug it, my face turned up to the sun like a hungry flower.

"The warmth is so amazing," I yelled to Veronica.

Veronica was a petite woman with almond-coloured eyes that sat above a smattering of freckles across her nose. Angry black stitches pulled the vertical gash on her arm together. Veronica had been forced into foster care during the Sixties Scoop, the large-scale removal of Indigenous children from their homes by the government's assimilationist child welfare system. She couldn't remember her birth family but could remember the trauma her white foster family put her through. Veronica was left to pay the price for all these white decisions, which is how she ended up in the hospital. Like Laurie, she had come straight to the open side of the ward from the emergency room and received privileges right away.

My first cigarette drag pulled me down to the freshly cut grass. "Wow," I said to no one in particular. "I can't remember the last time I had a head rush like this."

I smoked with my right hand and twisted blades of grass between my fingers with the other. I gulped back as much nicotine-tinged air as my lungs would take, pulling hard on the extra light cigarettes my grampa had given me during visiting hours.

Veronica plopped onto a patch of grass next to me. She squinted an eye against a plume of smoke that curled up from her cigarette.

I closed my eyes and listened to birds chirping in saplings that whipped in the wind from the traffic along the town's main thoroughfare. Veronica smacked my leg lightly to get my attention.

"Did I tell you what the nurse said to me this morning? She said I wasn't really trying to kill myself."

"What do you mean?" I sat up.

Veronica held up her wrist. "I bled through the bandage in the night so I took it off. I asked the nurse—I don't remember which one—if I could see a doctor about it. She blew me off. Told me it wasn't even a serious wound. She said that I obviously cut myself for attention. I thought I cut deep enough."

I apologized to Veronica. "I'm starting to realize it's not about getting better in here," I said. "It's all about following the rules. Whoever does it best is discharged. The people who try to fight back get stuck."

"Break's up, ladies," Laurie called to us. "Time to go back in."

"Already?" I asked.

✳

My assigned psychiatrist returned from his summer vacation. A few days later, we met in a cramped room with a window. The sun shone right into my eye, and part of me wondered if the psychiatrist had asked me to sit in this chair as some sort of psychological test. The psychiatrist was a slight man with scraggly eyebrows that took up too much real estate on his face. He frowned at my file and asked if I wanted to leave. I told him I did, badly. Since they needed the free bed, he said he'd discharge me if I promised to follow up with my psychologist in the city. I didn't tell him I didn't have a psychologist, just a drug counsellor my university had referred me to. I walked out of the ward with yellow carbon copies of my discharge papers and a month's supply of my medication.

It took five years for the world to drop dead again. Half-empty packages of cold medicine, expired Tylenol, a bottle of Midol, boxes of allergy medicine, and my sharpest knives were scattered across my tiled bathroom floor. I had promised my partner I would get rid of my stash, but the pills—white, blue, yellow, orange, and some with letters or lines pressed into their faces—had whispered so seductively to me that I should keep them. Forty-six pills in total, but was it enough?

In the five years since my last inpatient hospitalization, I had graduated from university with a journalism degree and began a career in literary events after the antipsychotics I was prescribed during my first hospitalization stole my ability to write. I waded into a healthy relationship. In the wider world, the Zika virus broke out, the Panama Papers were published, Donald Trump was trying to become president, and a gorilla named Harambè was shot and killed at a Cincinnati zoo.

After my close call in the bathroom, I had insisted on walking to the hospital with my partner, M. I needed, somehow, to prolong the time between resigning myself to inpatient psychiatric help and actually being admitted. Rain fell horizontally and bit at our faces. I focused on my feet moving forward and retreated inward, seeing but not really seeing the post-war bungalows we passed, the vintage walk-ups, the slick black tree branches grasping for the sky.

"You can thank Howard Hughes for the beds," my partner, M., had told me in the emergency room. "He got in a plane crash or something and had to be hospitalized. He was so badly injured and uncomfortable in his hospital bed that he had his engineers sent to his room. When they got there, he told them, 'You need to make a new bed for me and everyone in here.'"

Well, thanks, Howard Hughes. Your bed was the least broken thing on the open side of the psych ward. With the top of the hospital bed propped up, I could see out the window, which surveyed the city's east end. It was grey and foggy. The buildings on the horizon were shadows of themselves. Everything else was brown and muddy, though I had noticed the odd tiny green bud bursting from the tips of branches during the tempestuous walk to the hospital.

An old woman in the bed next to mine slept with her mouth open. Snores rattled through her chapped lips. A speaker between the two beds crackled, and a voice filled our room. "Attention, everyone, dinner is now being served. Please wash your hands and report to the dining room."

I passed a woman in the hallway who was talking to her yellowed toenails. She rocked back and forth and listed names to her feet in a Greek accent. "Constantine, Nicholas, Maximus, Agatha."

The psych ward in the city was dingier than the one in the suburbs. In the dining area, a torn orange pleather couch watched the evening news. There was a fist-sized crater in the wall next to the television.

"Patience, all you boys lack patience," a stout man in a hospital gown said. I pulled out a chair at his table. "You're too eager to attack, and it's your downfall."

"I'm no boy, Hector," a middle-aged man with a lively dancing face said. "And I'll whip your ass in chess anytime, old man."

A few giggles rose from the others at the table.

"Who are you?" a woman sitting next to me who used a wheelchair asked. I told her, and she introduced herself as June.

"Welcome," Hector said. "You play any chess?"

"A little," I said between mouthfuls of a cheese sandwich. The city hospital was better at providing a vegetarian diet.

"Don't change the subject," the lively faced man said. "I'm challenging you to a match, Hector."

"Please, Mark. The only one of you I actually want to play is Rodney, and he won't play me."

Rodney was a colossal man whose face sloped to one side, perhaps from a stroke. A spit bubble popped in the corner of his mouth when he spoke. "Can't sit still that long. Plus, you're a sore loser."

Mark jumped to his feet. "See?" he yelled to Hector. "I'm your only real competition here. Come on."

"After supper, Mark."

Mark sucked his teeth and slumped back into his seat.

"So, Miranda," Hector said. "Tell us a bit about yourself. How old are you? What do you do?"

I swallowed a lump of sandwich. I told the group that I was twenty-five and lived on the Danforth.

"You Greek?" Mark asked. He launched into rapid Greek I couldn't understand.

"No, but I was baptized Greek Orthodox. There were no Ukrainian churches where I lived."

"Didn't think so." Mark's face cracked into a smile. "Not with that light hair."

"What do you do for work?" Hector asked.

I paused. Was I still technically employed if I was existing in a place where time dropped dead? Would my position as an event manager still be available to me when my world started spinning again? Did I even still want it?

"I'm a writer," I said. It wasn't untrue. I had published the odd nonfiction piece here and there, but it hardly paid the bills.

A boy who had been ignoring his food to scribble in his notebook looked up at me.

"Is that so? I noticed you reading earlier," Hector said. "Would I know anything you've written?"

"No, but if you want any book recommendations, let me know."

I left the dining area to bus my tray. My roommate's dinner was there, untouched. "Can I bring her her food?" I asked a nurse with spiky hair and purple-rimmed glasses who was guarding the meals.

"Is it your tray?"

I explained that it was my roommate's and that I didn't want her to miss dinner.

"If she wants supper, she'll have to get out of bed."

"Isn't it more important that she eat something?" I asked. "I usually feel worse on an empty stomach."

The nurse lunged for the tray as if I was about to shoplift it. "She has to get it herself."

Later, I sat next to the pay phone in the dining area and fingered the graffiti on the wall. I listened to the line trill. People shuffled past me on their way to the decaf coffee machine. The answering machine hadn't had time to pick up when a woman in a peach dress with blood-red blooms walked by and farted right in my face. Definitely back in the ward.

*

A nurse led me into a quiet room off the open side's main hallway. The room was in better condition than most here. There were limited scratches, the seating was mismatched but unscarred, and there was only one small dent in the wall. It smelled like everywhere else in the ward, though—lingering disinfectant mingled with piss and shit in recycled air.

The psychiatrist entered. He was an older man with a shock of salt-and-pepper hair, not so different from the admitting psychiatrist who had given me so much trouble during my first hospitalization. "I'm Dr. Martin." He reached out and shook my hand. His was fleshy and warm. It was the first time I had dared to touch a psych ward doctor.

"Why don't you tell me a bit about what brought you in yesterday?" he asked.

When a person is admitted to a hospital's psychiatric unit, they have to tell the same story over and over. To the triage nurse, to the emergency room physician, to the on-call psychiatrist, to the medical doctor in the ward, to the assigned nurse, and to the assigned psychiatrist. By the time I was faced with Dr. Martin, I only had the energy for the abridged version.

My grandfather had died of a brain bleed two years ago—the

closest person I'd had to a father, the only man in my family who had loved me unconditionally since birth. My stepdad's father was diagnosed with stage 4 cancer the following summer. To avoid the hole one grandfather's absence created, and in anticipation of the second opening me up like an autopsy, I threw myself into my job and side hustles until one-hundred-hour workweeks became the norm.

"I don't have a lot of people fighting in my corner," I explained. "My grandfather always did. He's the first person I want to talk to when I do well at work, read a good book, or luck into some money. The combination of losing him, preparing to lose my remaining grandfather, and the stress of working so much put me in a dark spot."

Dr. Martin thanked me for my honesty. He told me I was in the right place. He was going to work on helping me feel safe while I was in the hospital.

"Speaking of"—I finally came to what I saw as the point of the conversation—"am I still formed?"

"At this point, yes," he said. "You're still on a seventy-two-hour hold, but given your eloquence, I won't sign a Form 3 once it expires. You'll be here voluntarily."

The interview was going well. I pushed harder and asked about privileges.

"I'll tell the nurse you can wear your street clothes," he said. "Let's leave the rest until tomorrow. I think you'll do fine on a pass, but I want to make sure you're feeling nice and safe first."

Dr. Martin stood and shook my hand again. It was frighteningly human. The warmth lingered after he let go. He held the door open for me and told me what a strong and capable woman I was.

*

I sat on the hallway floor with Nick, the boy who had been busy with his notebook during that first meal, and Tim, who had approached me in the hallway after my meeting with the psychiatrist to give me two drawings with his Instagram handle where the artist's signature normally goes.

"Yo, that short lady who was admitted today trips me out. The fucking angels shit. I wasn't trying to be rude she was just, like, fucking getting in my head," Tim said. He was in a mix of hospital and street clothes, as if he was wearing everything he owned to try to make himself seem bigger. His face hovered so close to the drawing that he was bent over that his nose almost scraped the page.

"Try not to let it bother you," I said. Nick and I were doing low-impact yoga on the linoleum. I pushed out thoughts of all the rank bare feet that had walked across the floor. And who might have peed on it. "Nick, focus on your breathing. Deep and slow."

"Don't get me wrong," Tim continued. "I like her. Me and her daughter even went to the same school and shit. And it's not that I don't believe in angels. I just need to be in the right headspace to hear that, you know?"

Nick murmured a sound of agreement and winced when he rose over his outstretched leg. "Thanks for the stretches. I used to work in construction. That's how I fucked up my back."

Nick pushed his dreads back with a headband and told us about how much of an asshole his former boss was. He wouldn't go into all the details, but the guy owed Nick a lot of money and kept dodging him. One night, Nick showed up at his boss's house to collect.

"Craziest thing is, when I got inside, this guy had a pot-belly pig in his living room."

"You should've stolen it," I said. "And held it for ransom." Our laughter echoed through the blemished halls.

That night, I gathered with a few others in front of the news. Bernie Sanders had won Indiana. June and I watched Ted Cruz's concession speech. She said of Trump, simply, "His hair is so yellow."

The people in the ward, for the most part, greeted reminders of the outside world with a disinterested glance. It was easy to slip into a ward mentality—the nurses' fishbowl-like office was a constant reflection of the atmosphere. There was rarely a line to use the phone. The television often played the news, but it usually just provoked conspiracy theories or irrational rants. Despite a general eagerness to be discharged, most of us were hesitant to stay in touch with the world's rhythms. In a place where time dropped dead, it was easy to get caught up in the ward's machinations, in the slights, the tears, and the terrors of other people who drifted through the halls. The hospital became our only reality.

I lined up at the nurses' station to collect my morning meds. I gave my name at a window fitted with an intercom like at a bus station. The nurse slid my pills through the slot in a small paper cup. I was about to throw them back when I noticed they looked different from my usual pills. They were orange and elongated. Mine were white and round.

"These aren't my meds," I said.

"Yes, they are," the nurse said.

"This doesn't look like Klonopin. And where's my Lexapro?"

"Those meds are what's on your chart. I think I would know better than you would. Take them so the next person can get their meds."

"I'm not taking them," I said.

I could see through the nurses' station into the locked side of the ward, where Yolanda, a girl who was briefly on open, lined up for her pills. She swallowed what I expected were my meds. "Seriously," I said. "I think you gave me Yolanda's meds." I pointed through the glass.

The nurse sighed. "Do I need to get your psychiatrist?"

I told her to go ahead. While we waited, she doled out meds to the next patient, and the next, and the next.

Early research noted that people with BPD who were hospitalized had a tendency to create disruptive emotional conflicts between hospital staff. I was willing to pit hospital staff against one another if they made mistakes that interfered with my health. A person with limited agency has to use whatever tools are at their disposal to advocate for their wellness because no one is considered less trustworthy than a psychiatric patient. Except, perhaps, a psychiatric patient with BPD. The *Harvard Review of Psychiatry* article notes that people with BPD "were more likely to be described as 'manipulative, difficult to manage, unlikely to arouse sympathy, annoying, and not deserving of [health care] resources.'"

"She won't take her meds," the nurse said when Dr. Martin arrived.

"Dr. Martin," I said in my sweetest voice. "These aren't my meds." I tipped the paper cup to show him my pills. He glanced at my chart.

"She's right," he said. "This isn't her medication."

*

"You disappear and everything goes to shit," Nick said. We were out for a smoke after my first day pass. "And I'm like, 'Where's Miranda?'"

I had been back home on my three-hour pass when Hector showed June his balls. He only wore a hospital gown, always went commando, and apparently his testicles appreciated an audience. Hector was sent to lockdown.

I shook away the thought and blew a long stream of purplish smoke toward Coxwell Avenue. The third smoke break of the day coincided with recess across the street.

"Why would they put an elementary school so close to a hospital?" I asked.

Nick laughed. "Yeah, they didn't account for us, did they?"

Back upstairs, Hector was already back in open and dozing at a dining table. June was sitting in front of the television in her wheelchair. She watched Sean Connery lilt his way through a daytime movie. Nick was called away for a meeting with his doctor.

"You okay?" I sat on the squeaky leather sofa next to June. "I heard what happened."

"I'm having a bad day, hon." June's eyes were puffed and bloodshot. Her long hair lay on her back in tangles. "My social worker told my doctor I've been abusing painkillers. The fucking bitch. Now they're saying they're going to take them away."

I took June's hand in mine. Her eyes welled up.

"Did I ever tell you how I got into my wheelchair?" She squeezed my palm. Two of her children had died on the same day in separate incidents. "It was too much. I tried to kill myself. It didn't work. I was in a coma for two weeks and have been in crippling pain ever since. And now they want to take my meds away."

In the ward, as is the case with many institutional settings, an us-versus-them attitude pervaded, with *them* representing any figure of authority. This pervasive power dynamic pitted the patient against the doctor, which wasn't conducive to healing. But the psychiatric intensive care unit was where all sense of logic dropped dead. I could only say what I found myself saying over and over in the hospital. "I'm so sorry that happened to you."

Nick returned swearing. More bad news. Legal trouble from the encounter with the pot-belly pig.

Most of my friends on the ward were gathered in the dining room when I got back from my pass. They all cheered when I presented a box of Timbits. It almost felt like a homecoming.

"Where's Tim?" I asked Rodney, who munched on a honey-glazed. "I have something for him."

"In his room, I think." Rodney sprayed a few donut crumbs as he answered. I popped a chocolate Timbit in my mouth and headed to Tim's room.

Tim had asked me to get a plastic sleeve for a photo during my pass. He wanted it to protect a picture of his mother, who died a few years ago. When I got to his room, he was drawing in his bed.

"Hey." He took his headphones off. His tone was icy. "What do you want?"

"Can I come in? I brought you something."

He motioned me in. I dropped the photo in its sleeve on his bed. He looked at it briefly and then went back to drawing.

"Everything okay?" I asked.

"Yep." He put his headphones back on.

※

That night, Nick and I sat in what was called the South Lounge. It was where one of the ward pay phones and a foosball table with no ball lived. It was also where I had once heard Mark whisper loving words to his girlfriend only to scream *slut* at the phone after he banged it into the receiver.

"Honestly, fuck Tim," Nick said. "He's disrespectful as fuck."

During the Raptors game, with everyone gathered in front of the TV, Tim had called me a fucking bitch. My stomach had bottomed out, and my face had grown as hot as a fire poker.

"I know. You're right," I said and wiped some tears back. "I just don't understand why he would treat me this way. I've only ever been pleasant to him."

"He's just a shady guy." Nick's eyes were big and worried behind his glasses. "Sooner or later, he was going to snap. You're just today's target. I know he's been up in here stealing, causing all sorts of shit because he thinks it's funny. He drops the n-word around me to try to get a rise out of me. He's immature."

"I just want to go home."

"I know," Nick said. "But if I'm getting out of here tomorrow, you can't be far behind me. Patience. Play by their rules. Remember? You're the one who taught me that."

I was about to smile when Tim stalked by the windowed South Lounge, with something in his hand. He smacked my journal, which I kept in my room, against the glass windows, its insides revealed. He took a big swig from a bottle of Gatorade he had also stolen from me.

I wanted to tear the flesh off his face with my bare hands. I wanted to swear and stomp and destroy him because I had been kind to him. Because he had violated my trust. Because I had been having a good day before his bullshit.

Tim screamed and made for one of two doors that led into the lounge. Nick and I rushed to opposite doors, but I reached the one Tim made for. The door swung inward and hit me in the face. I shouldered it shut before Tim could slip in. Nick threw his weight against the other door so no matter how hard Tim pushed, he couldn't open it.

Nurses' soft-soled shoes squeaked down the hall. A doctor's dress shoes clicked behind. They surrounded Tim and pulled him from the door.

"He went into my room!" I yelled through the glass. "He stole my stuff!"

"That bitch took two of my drawings." Tim's face twisted in fury. He tried to wrestle free from the arms containing him. "I was just getting them back."

"Liar!" I screamed.

Nick vouched for me. A group of nurses and a doctor jostled Tim back to his room. The remaining nurse told me it was best to go back to mine too. She'd see to it that my journal was returned.

Later, I was reading in my bed when I heard a Ping-Pong ball bounce beyond my door. Then a hesitant knock. I raced over to hold it shut. There were no locks to protect me.

"Tim's here to apologize," Rodney said through the door. "And I'm here to snap him in two if he tries anything funny."

"Yo," Tim said. "Can we talk?"

I opened the door slightly and peeked through the crack.

"I'm sorry. You know I fucking love you." The cluck of the bouncing Ping-Pong ball peppered the apology.

"You don't treat people who you love like that. And besides, I have a boyfriend."

"I know. I was angry and jealous, I guess. I don't know. It was a fucked-up day."

I tersely thanked Tim for his apology and closed my door. The Ping-Pong ball's bouncing persisted. I fell asleep with my back wedged against the door. Just in case.

Tim had made me into a stereotype. I was trying so hard to navigate the ward in a smarter and less emotional manner during my second hospitalization. Instead, I felt like I embodied a 2009 investigation about clinicians' experiences working with people with BPD that reported that we have poor coping skills, present ongoing crisis behaviours, and have trouble interacting appropriately with others.

✳

By the next morning, Nick, Mark, and June had been discharged. "Let's go for a walk," Rodney said once I returned from the day's first smoke break. "The little monkey has been hiding from us."

I took it he meant Tim. We walked toward his room around the corner from the South Lounge. A moment of silence passed between us. "He's just a stupid kid, you know," Rodney said.

"That's no excuse."

"His brother was supposed to visit and didn't show up. I think he was upset."

There was no sign of Tim in the South Lounge.

"I'm not saying what he did was right," Rodney said. "But he's a mixed-up kid."

"We're all mixed up," I said. "I don't deserve to be the target of Tim's rage."

Tim's room was empty and his bed was pristine, unslept in.

We lingered in the eastern hallway and peered through the glass door separating the psych ward's locked side from open.

"The little monkey was raising hell last night," Rodney said. We headed toward the nurses' station.

"He was?" I felt my pulse quicken. For Rodney, this was a mission of caring. For me, it was more about figuring out where Tim was so I could shore up my defences.

"Splashing coffee all over the walls, cursing, and yelling."

We drifted past the interview rooms, but they were all empty. We continued back to the dining area, where Hector was reading the paper and a few other people were watching television and eating breakfast. No sign of Tim.

"Let's keep walking until we find him," Rodney said.

In the hallway, the Greek woman was out of her room and holding a conversation with her toes again. The back of her hospital gown was open, but I suspected she had bigger things to worry about than Rodney and I noticing the twisted strap of her nude-coloured bra.

"They probably gave him a shot." Rodney wiped away a fleck of the spit gathered in the corner of his mouth. "They did that to me once."

We looped around the nurses' station to another door that looked into the locked ward.

"Yep, there's the little monkey." Rodney pointed through the glass.

Tim was locked away. Asleep on a cot in the hallway.

"Went too wild and got the needle," Rodney said.

At lunch, I sat at a dining table with Rodney and Hector, who laughed about Tim's late-night escapades. I opened my journal to write. I flipped to find a fresh page but instead found the word *bitch* scrawled by Tim in capital letters. It was on the next page. And the next one too. Pages and pages of angrier and angrier versions of the word *bitch*. I ripped out each ruined page, one by one.

"I want to go home," I said to Dr. Martin as soon as he arrived for our appointment.

His face dropped as if he'd miss me if I left. "I'm not sure that's the best thing for you right now."

"I'm here voluntarily," I reminded him. "And I don't feel safe anymore. I think I've gotten all I can from my time here. As you know, I've already arranged follow-up outpatient counselling. I think it's time for me to transition."

Before I came to the hospital, I had put my name on a waitlist for free therapy provided by a community-based social services agency. Based on my last hospitalization experience, I knew there might not be many outpatient supports available, and I wasn't going to avoid mental health care for another five years until I found myself in crisis again. I wanted this hospital stay to be the last time I was considered too much of a danger to myself to make my own decisions.

I scooched my chair a little closer to his. In psychoanalysis, there's a term for when a therapist's feelings, emotions, and values are activated by identifying with their patient's experiences—countertransference. Countertransference is common but becomes problematic if it leads to harmful or unethical behaviours, or negatively affects the therapeutic relationship.

"What if I increase your passes to six hours? Will you stay a little longer?" Dr. Martin asked. His eyes gleamed with what I perceived to be hope.

I had already started to suspect countertransference was happening. During one session, Dr. Martin likened my circumstances to that of a recent immigrant after I described how overwhelmed I felt trying to take care of myself. He explained that I had no social support net to catch me if I fell. I was on my own. His university degree from a European medical school hung on the wall.

I was flattered that Dr. Martin saw some of his own struggles in mine. I appreciated his empathy, but that wasn't my reality. My family was geographically accessible. My grandparents and my mother did their best to help me when I stumbled. Even if my theory of countertransference was merely paranoia or hypervigilance, how could he help me if he didn't really see me for who I was?

The base of my neck tingled. A gentle queasiness disturbed my stomach. I don't think anyone can say with any certainty if another person is attracted to them unless it's explicitly communicated. But there are clues—the way their eyes light up, the quest for common ground, the excuse for proximity. Dr. Martin had been kind to me, but after my first hospitalization, I didn't trust male doctors charged with my care.

And I had good reason not to. Early research portrayed people with BPD as so enticing that they frequently seduced "even experienced therapists into serious boundary violations, including patient-therapist sex." People with the disorder weren't just blamed for our own lapses in acceptable functioning. We were blamed for clinicians' harmful behaviour too. There truly was no winning for people with BPD seeking treatment.

"After everything that happened with Tim, my anxiety would improve if I was discharged," I said. "Please, Dr. Martin?" I asked the question in my most cloying voice. If Dr. Martin was charmed by me on any level, I reasoned, maybe I could at least use it to my advantage.

"How about I give you a full day pass today and you give it one more night? Just come back to sleep here. We can revisit tomorrow, and if you're still feeling the same, we'll see about your discharge."

I took the pass. I didn't want to fracture the goodwill I'd culti-vated with Dr. Martin. I couldn't. I needed his affection in whatever form it came. He was the only person who could release me from the hospital.

✳

People with BPD are undoubtedly overrepresented in health care settings. It's thought that 10 per cent of psychiatric outpatients are diagnosed with BPD, and 20 per cent of inpatients have the dis-order. We have to keep returning to care because we're the least likely of all people to receive the help necessary to break the cycle. Instead of seeing people with BPD as irritating or burdensome, the medical community should utilize the high rates at which people with BPD seek treatment as an opportunity to learn more about the disorder and how to treat it. Research from 2015 showed that tar-geted intervention was successful at improving clinicians' attitudes toward people with the disorder. More helpful and empathetic treatment of people with BPD could go a long way in reducing re-institutionalization and promoting recovery.

The next morning, I sat in the South Lounge, the phone cradled on my shoulder. I yawned and shuddered. Rodney's prized gold chain was stolen yesterday. My eyes watered when I thought of Rodney's broad shoulders wracked with sobs so violent that he was sent to lockdown. I needed to get the hell out of this endless place. Only misery could foment in a space where there was such vast pur-poselessness, so little hope, nothing to look forward to.

The line connected. My partner's sleepy voice filled my ear.

"They're discharging me today."

"Want me to come pick you up?" M. asked.

"It's okay. Come over tonight."

A few hours later, I pushed through the hospital's revolving doors. My backpack was slung over one shoulder, filled with my clothes, books, meds, and my signed discharge papers. I sucked back the warm May air and squinted in the sunshine. I hustled away from the hospital, passing green lawns blossoming with cheerful flowers, walking the same route M. and I had taken weeks earlier. But the slick black boughs we had seen were filled with bright green leaves. Birds flitted from tree to tree and sang me home. During the time I was hospitalized, spring had bloomed in the city.

The world was born again.

FATALLY ATTRACTIVE

Composed and stern, attorney Camille Vasquez told the court that her client, actor Johnny Depp, had tried to leave the room anytime he and his then-wife, actor Amber Heard, got into a conflict. "But his trying to leave enraged Ms. Heard. She would resort to physical violence, throwing things at him, hitting him."

In 2018, Heard penned a *Washington Post* op-ed (with a helping hand from the American Civil Liberties Union), which detailed what it was like to be a victim of alleged domestic violence in the public arena. The implication that Depp was the perpetrator of that abuse, Depp's team of lawyers argued, was impossible to ignore. Hence, Heard had allegedly defamed him.

The words *borderline personality disorder* didn't appear in Vasquez's opening remarks. They didn't need to. Anyone who lived with the disorder could see what she was cueing up. Heard's frantic efforts to avoid real or perceived abandonment, as Vasquez described, is a diagnostic symptom of BPD.

These frantic efforts are among the behaviours that make people with BPD so grating to the general public, which contributes to BPD being the most stigmatized mental health condition. We're whirlwinds of instability, impulsivity, and intense and highly changeable emotions. Studies show that the disorder is hard to understand and the least likely of all mental illnesses to provoke sympathy from the average person. Depp's lawyers understood the inherent power of Hollywood storytelling—the good guy overcoming impossible odds to defeat a villain. His legal team took advantage of public sentiment toward BPD to argue that Heard was the primary abuser in their relationship and had defamed Depp when she implied the opposite in her op-ed.

The first time BPD was mentioned in more than passing or inference was on the tenth day of the trial when clinical and forensic psychologist Shannon Curry took the stand for Depp's camp. She told the court she suspected that Heard had BPD. "[People with BPD] can react violently, they can react aggressively. They will often physically prevent their partner from trying to leave if their partner wants to get space from all of this intense emotion. And oftentimes, they will be abusive to their partners in these situations," Curry said. "People with [BPD], it seems to be a predictive factor for women who implement violence against their partner."

Depp's legal team relied on BPD to do the heavy lifting in positioning Heard as an abuser. But numerous studies demonstrate that a BPD diagnosis alone does not predict violent behaviour. Instead, co-occurring diagnoses like substance use disorder, antisocial personality disorder, or childhood abuse raise the risk a person will commit violent acts. People with BPD, like most people with serious mental illnesses, are far more likely to be the victims of violence than the perpetrators. One study found that nearly half of all people with BPD experience violence in adulthood. Much of that violence—88 per cent—comes in the form of a physically abusive partner.

Unfortunately, Depp's legal team and witnesses weren't the first to perpetuate the notion that women with BPD are conniving manipulators with violent tendencies. The media had been doing it for decades.

"I never saw her as a villain," Glenn Close explained of her portrayal of Alex Forrest in the 1987 film *Fatal Attraction*, during an interview with *ABC News*. "I always thought she was a human being in a lot of pain, and she needed a lot of help."

Fatal Attraction follows the fallout from a weekend-long extramarital affair between Close's troubled character and Dan Gallagher, played by Michael Douglas. Forrest's mental illness isn't made explicit in the film; however, her behaviour is so synonymous with BPD that a professor once told Close he used the character as an extreme example of the disorder.

Fatal Attraction was likely the first and certainly the most prominent movie to so firmly place a woman with BPD in the role of the bad guy. Close's Forrest is initially alluring, the ultimate femme fatale, but over the course of her entanglement with Gallagher, the layers of her charm are stripped away. This depiction aligns with mirroring or masking, a strategy people with BPD use in which they embody the characteristics or whims of a desired person to feel closer to them. But as the story unfolds, Forrest is revealed to be an aggressive woman who self-harms when deserted, stalks her paramour, boils a family pet, and kidnaps a child in an attempt to get a man to take responsibility for his actions. Director Adrian Lyne pushed BPD symptomology to such extremes in *Fatal Attraction* that it surely influenced public perception of the disorder. A *Los Angeles Times* review of the film, which called it "the most talked-about movie" released that year and touched on its anti-feminist message, described Californian audiences who hissed and booed at Close's gruesome scenes.

The climax sees a pregnant Forrest murdered in self-defence by Gallagher's wife, Beth (Anne Archer), after Forrest breaks into their home and attacks the couple. Lyne did a great disservice to women with BPD throughout the film, but it isn't until its very end that Forrest becomes explicitly violent toward the Gallagher family— a last-minute change Close protested for weeks. (The original ending of the film had Forrest die by suicide, with Gallagher framed for her death.) It's Gallagher who commits the initial act of brutality when he chokes Forrest in her apartment, an act the viewer watches through her eyes. Yet, the audience is still meant to root for him.

Forrest is meant to be the most frightening part of the film, but it's the idea that I deserve to die if my illness deteriorates enough that terrifies me.

The crowd reaction to Forrest in *Fatal Attraction* was echoed in the general public's treatment of Heard during the defamation trial. By the time it started, there was already plenty of evidence of Depp's capacity for destructive acts memorialized online. Photos of Depp's blood, Heard's lipstick, and black paint smeared on the mirrors of their destroyed Australian rental mansion. Heard's bare face with an alleged bruise that sat high on her pale cheekbone. Screenshots of text messages Depp exchanged with Paul Bettany about murdering Heard and fucking her corpse. Reports from the libel trial Depp lost in London, England, that he had head-butted Heard in the face. But, in the U.S. defamation suit, the audience was still rooting for Depp.

Depp's fans showed up in hordes online and outside the courtroom. Reports described people who flew in from overseas to stand outside the Fairfax Circuit Court. People lined up as early as one in the morning to secure passes to the proceedings and slept in their cars to save money on accommodations. The amount of online vitriol Heard was subject to during the defamation trial was astounding. At times, it felt as deafening as pro-Trump posts in 2016. (Depp enlisted Adam Waldman, a lawyer with ties to Russian oligarch Oleg Deripaska, who worked with the Trump campaign.) In what would later be dubbed as "one of the worst cases of platform manipulation," by a research firm hired by Heard, hashtags that referred to Heard as a turd, a liar, and a monster overwhelmed TikTok and Twitter (and the online pile-on continued for months after the trial). A social media expert who testified for Heard found over one million negative posts about the actor. Both Heard and her infant daughter received death threats.

I'd hazard a guess that Heard likely felt very unsafe during much of the trial. But it's people with BPD who are typically thought of as dangerous. It could stem from an ambiguous symptom of the disorder. People with BPD tend to engage in impulsive and occasionally unpredictable behaviours. These behaviours, which include reckless spending, gambling, or substance use, tend to be more damaging to individuals with BPD, though they can affect their loved ones. More likely, it's the connection between female criminality and BPD that sustains the stereotype. Aileen Wuornos, who confessed to seven murders; Alyssa Bustamante, a fifteen-year-old who murdered her nine-year-old neighbour; and Elizabeth Wettlaufer, one of Canada's worst serial killers, were all publicly linked with the disorder. Wuornos met the criteria for BPD, but she was also diagnosed with a psychopathic personality, antisocial personality disorder, and had a horrifying childhood, which professionals believed played a large role in her criminal behaviour. Bustamante suffered from major depression and displayed certain features of BPD, such as self-harm and suicide attempts. But mental health professionals at her trial testified that she showed early signs of bipolar disorder. Her attorneys presented evidence that her Prozac dose, which was increased two weeks prior to the murder, could have been a factor that contributed to Bustamante's crime. Wettlaufer, a registered nurse who killed her patients, was struggling with a long-term addiction to opioids and prescription medication. She was diagnosed with obsessive-compulsive disorder and depression when she committed the murders, and she had been taking the antipsychotic Seroquel, which can increase violent feelings in some people. There's no doubt people with BPD, like any human beings, are capable of violence. But there's usually a lot more at play than a BPD diagnosis.

Perhaps the most notorious fictional female criminal with BPD is Livia Soprano (Nancy Marchand). *The Sopranos* follows Tony Soprano (James Gandolfini), a New Jersey mob boss struggling with malaise and the idea he got involved with the mafia during its death rattle instead of its golden years. Of course, any Italian man worth his weight is nothing without his family, and Tony's loved ones play large roles in his life. No one casts a greater shadow than his mother, Livia. She's alienated all of her children with her ferocious guilt trips save for Tony, which leaves him as her primary caregiver. Tony puts Livia in a nursing home against her wishes after she starts a kitchen fire because she's preoccupied with spying on her neighbours, which creates a fatal fracture in their overwrought relationship. During a therapy session, Tony's psychiatrist Dr. Melfi (Lorraine Bracco) suggests that his mother might be behind a recent assassination attempt on his life—and she's right—and diagnoses Livia with BPD. "These people have no love or compassion," Melfi says before Tony launches himself across the room to attack her.

Like Close's Forrest, Marchand's Livia routinely made top villain lists. But Marchand's portrayal of the disorder rang truer for me—to the point I often couldn't understand why she was considered so villainous. People with BPD are known for having unusual or "primitive" defence mechanisms, which serve an important role in getting their needs met. Marchand's Livia hones these mechanisms into an art form. Livia could never be a part of the family business; the mafia is a patriarchal organization. But through her manipulation of Tony and his uncle Junior (Dominic Chianese), Livia plays a major role in the family's operations from her nursing home. She uses every piece of information that comes her way as a weapon. She has to. She's a woman in a man's world who uses the power she has to get her needs met, no matter how skewed those needs may be.

Unfortunately, *The Sopranos* also depicted a woman with BPD as capable of inflicting massive amounts of physical and emotional violence with none of the empathy, remorse, or guilt so frequently found in people with the disorder. A recent study confirmed women with BPD experience higher levels of shame, guilt, and fear than healthy female controls. The disorder is painful to live with. But thanks to media portrayals, the myth that people with BPD don't experience remorse persists. As Tony would say, "It's a stereotype, and it's offensive."

That Heard didn't show enough remorse during her testimony was one of the criticisms lobbed at the actor by print and social media. But Heard was far from an ideal victim even if she had been more apologetic. The money from her divorce settlement that Heard had pledged to charities didn't materialize in full. She readily admitted to calling Depp belittling names and hitting him in self-defence. A marriage counsellor who worked with the couple testified that Depp and Heard's dynamic was one of mutual abuse. Depp fans dredged up Heard's 2009 arrest for striking her girlfriend at the time, Tasya van Ree, who called reporting about the incident misrepresentative.

Depp had his own demons. He admitted to using drugs and alcohol to self-medicate and numb his pain, though testified that Heard's characterization of his substance use was "grossly embellished." Photographs entered into evidence showed huge bags of pot in Depp's recording studio and four lines of coke neatly cut on a glass table accompanied by a tampon applicator—a method for snorting coke that Heard said her sister had taught Depp. There was also the widely shared photo of Depp passed out, one of several like it, with his head thrown back into a bunch of pillows, while a spilled ice cream container melted on his crossed legs. Unsealed pretrial documents revealed that Ellen Barkin, who was in a brief relationship with Depp in the late nineties, called the actor "controlling" and "jealous." She alleged he had once thrown a wine bottle across a room in her direction.

Both parties were complicated individuals with signs of mental illness. What was interesting to me was that Depp's disorder didn't receive a fraction of the hatred Heard was subject to online. Substance use disorder is more widespread than BPD and perhaps as a result more relatable. This could also be why Heard didn't identify with a BPD diagnosis. Psychologist Dawn Hughes testified for Heard that she thought the actor had post-traumatic stress disorder brought on by intimate partner violence. In the murky he-said-she-said soup that was the defamation trial, one thing was clear: PTSD and substance use disorder were viewed as more sympathetic and manageable diagnoses by both clinicians and the general public.

But BPD and PTSD share many similarities and commonly co-occur (including in yours truly). Both diagnoses are characterized by difficulties with emotional regulation, mood swings, episodes of anger, and dissociation. Complex PTSD, or C-PTSD, which can occur when a person experiences repeated or prolonged trauma, has long been proposed as an alternative diagnosis to BPD. Many clinicians view it as a more accurate and less stigmatizing label.

But it was easier for trial watchers to reconcile a BPD diagnosis with the monster they wanted Heard to be. One Reddit user believed Heard was "lying" and "claiming victimhood." The user wrote that they had been married to two women with BPD (though conceded only one ex-wife was actually diagnosed with the disorder) and believed Heard was demonstrating an "abusive relationship cycle" that all people with BPD engage in. Heard's allegations, the Reddit user believed, were simply part of a "smear campaign."

There is no link between BPD and dishonesty. I believe that people with BPD are no more deceptive than the average person, though perhaps they lie for different reasons, like to prevent abandonment. But there are pages upon pages of pop psychology websites that insist people with BPD not only lie but that our illness causes us to believe our own lies. I can find two possible origins of this myth: the first is a single study published in 1986 in which the author described four cases of people with BPD who were pathological liars. The second is one of the most stigmatizing books ever written about the disorder, *Stop Walking on Eggshells: Taking Your Life Back When Someone You Care About Has Borderline Personality Disorder* by Paul T. Mason and Randi Kreger. "People with BPD are fully convinced their skewed feelings and beliefs—be they positive or negative—are unquestionably true," the authors wrote. This opinion, which has been repeated ad nauseam, invalidates people with BPD's experiences. It makes it easier for others to discount us when we're victimized. It gaslights people with the disorder.

Around the time Heard and Depp began dating, I was in my own tempestuous relationship and going through my own trial. Like Heard, I was trying to convince an audience (albeit a much smaller one) that my unusual behaviour—the constant crying, self-harm, inability to maintain important relationships, and substance abuse—stemmed from the impacts of early childhood trauma and not a penchant for dramatics and misbehaviour. But, like Heard, I had a relatability problem. Few people believed my allegations.

"Are you sure your stepdad hurt you when you were a kid?" the guy I dated in university asked after he met my family for the first time. I had surmised a statement to this effect was coming. My boyfriend had spent most of the afternoon laughing at my stepdad's jokes and shooting pool with him in my grandparents' basement. "He seems so friendly."

A downpour of tears burst from me. I buried my head into my pillow in the bedroom of my apartment in Toronto's Gay Village. Between howls, I tried to explain that there was a side of my stepdad that my boyfriend didn't see. A side that very few people saw. It was a frightening side exasperated by physical pain and addiction. His mood could change from sunny to stormy in a flash. Like Heard explained when she testified, I had to get good at paying attention to the different versions of him if I wanted to avoid harm.

I didn't have to convince the world that Captain Jack Sparrow was capable of violent acts. I only had to convince my loved ones that a disabled man with his own demons was too rough with his behaviourally challenged stepdaughter.

"Was it really that bad? Or were you blowing it out of proportion?" my boyfriend asked. "You do sometimes make a bigger deal out of things than you need to."

This remark provoked more tears, which led to one of our frequent fights. Our conflicts were protracted and intense. They lasted hours before they sputtered out, only to brew up again days later. The details of the fight on that night are murky, but I imagine I accused my partner of "being mean," the only shorthand I had at the time for feeling invalidated. He was ferociously stubborn, a pedantic student, and probably replied that a family member had also told him my allegations weren't true.

"How could you trust my family over me?" I would have cried. "All they've done is ruin my life!"

My boyfriend probably pointed out that I was exaggerating at that very moment. And the fight would have motored forward and made familiar detours like threats to leave if I self-harmed again— the only tool my partner had for dealing with my scarier symptoms, undiagnosed at the time. We'd argue about how much makeup I wore, that my part-time profession as a weed dealer was unladylike, that my emotions and past were "too real" for my boyfriend to handle until we forgot what we were fighting about in the first place. We brought out the worst in each other.

For me, "the worst" was the only time in my adult life I was physically aggressive toward a loved one. During a similarly dismal evening, when it was cold enough for our breath to linger in the air outside, we argued in an alley near Bathurst subway station. I didn't have the tools to deal with the sorrow that flooded me when my boyfriend implied that I wasn't good enough for him. He turned to walk into the night.

Growing up, my stepdad had taught my brother and me that the only way to deal with people who disrespected you was "to give them a good pounding." I heard the scream tear from my throat and watched from outside my body as I raced toward my boyfriend and closed the distance between us. I pulled my hand into a fist, just the way my stepdad taught me, and let it fly toward his face. The weight of what was about to happen brought me back into my body with the force of a punch. I tried to stop. I pulled my fist back, but it hooked his shoulder.

"Did you actually just fucking hit me?" My partner's face was a mask of shock and fury. "This is fucked."

"I'm so sorry." I dropped to my knees in the slush. I begged for him to forgive me and sobbed until my throat was raw. I was so ashamed that I had done the very thing that made me so frightened of my stepdad.

My boyfriend's moment of shame came later. I remember the pop his bones made as they broke on the arm of my couch when he punched it in frustration.

We stopped dating the summer before my final year of university. A few weeks later, I was hospitalized in inpatient psychiatric intensive care for the first time—another black mark against my crumbling credibility.

The undercurrent in many of the fights between me and my partner, and in the online comments about the defamation trial, centred on choice. Heard and I would be more sympathetic figures if we chose to get help for the symptoms of BPD. The idea that a mentally ill person is only worthy of empathy if they're in care implies the existence of a flawless psychiatric system that is easily accessible and equipped to treat people with BPD. This isn't the reality of mental health care in North America. BPD is a broad and poorly understood diagnosis. There are no pharmacological options available to treat the disorder (though many people with BPD take medication for comorbidities). There's only specialized, intensive, and long-term therapy that requires a team of clinicians whose availability and presence vary widely based on location. It can be traumatizing to receive help in inpatient care, where a person can be forcibly confined and medicated against their will. Even if the system was perfect and treatment was widespread and available, would the same level of contempt be directed toward a cancer patient who was pre-treatment? Or one who declined treatment? Agency is vital to people with chronic illnesses. People with BPD shouldn't be the exception.

People with BPD have been wrestling with the misconception that they choose to be ill or exaggerate their symptoms since the disorder was first recognized in the 1930s. *Girl, Interrupted* brought this falsehood to the general public's attention. Released in 1999, the film is based on the real-life story of Susanna Kaysen's extended stay at McLean Hospital where she was diagnosed with BPD. The film opens when Kaysen (Winona Ryder) tries to die by suicide. It follows her into a private and well-funded psychiatric hospital where she's admitted against her will. During her time in the hospital, Kaysen meditates on the nature of sanity, befriends her fellow patients, and even comes to rely on her surroundings.

After a tumultuous escape from the hospital with fellow patient Lisa (Angelina Jolie), who pushes former patient Daisy (Brittany Murphy) to suicide, Kaysen returns to the ward worse off than ever. She has a vile and racist confrontation with Nurse Valerie (Whoopi Goldberg), who tells her, "You're not crazy. You're a lazy, self-indulgent girl who is driving herself crazy!" This echoes an earlier conversation with Kaysen's love interest and one with her psychologist, Dr. Wick (Vanessa Redgrave), in which she asks Kaysen if she's willing to commit herself to the hospital for life in the name of indulging her flaws. Kaysen spends the rest of the movie buckling down, taking her meds, actively participating in therapy, and writing until she's recovered enough to be released. The thrust of the film suggests that Susanna was allowing her BPD to debilitate her. Unlike the rest of the women in the ward, she had the agency and intelligence all along to merely will her illness away through enough cognitive effort. This insult actively harms women with BPD who face considerable stigma from the medical industry when and if they reach out for help.

One Reddit user who was watching the Depp-Heard defamation trial likened BPD to a death sentence—not for people with the disorder but for those around them. They alleged many people kill themselves to escape abusive partners with BPD or are murdered by their spouses with BPD "in a fit of rage." (I was unable to find any evidence of either allegation.) The Reddit user, presumably referring to Heard, wrote it was time to "grow up, take accountability," and stop playing the victim. Accountability was at the centre of both sides' closing arguments in the trial. Both asked the jury to hold the actors accountable for their behaviour. Online, it was Heard who was often beseeched to get help for BPD. Depp's substance abuse issues didn't provoke the same pleas for intervention.

Early into Heard's testimony about her volatile relationship with Depp, I attended Yale University and the National Education Alliance for Borderline Personality Disorder's annual conference. The timely virtual event was to focus on themes of disruptive behaviours. Two keynote speeches were planned: former NFL receiver Brandon Marshall was to speak about his experience living with the disorder, and psychologist Alan E. Fruzzetti was to present the clinical keynote.

I was more interested in Fruzzetti's presentation. I already knew what life with BPD felt like. I wanted to learn what clinical advancements were in development to help people live better with the disorder. But Fruzzetti's keynote wasn't for people with BPD; it was about us. His presentation, "The Impact of Suicide Attempts and Self-Harm on Family Members," covered five common problems experienced by family members of people with BPD who are suicidal or engage in non-suicidal self-injury. I made it to the third problem— the stigma family members experience when they have a loved one who is suicidal—before I slammed my laptop shut in anger.

It's important to advocate for informed support networks, but the keynote reinforced a stereotype that runs through so many pop culture characterizations of BPD: that the biggest burden of the disorder is the unreasonable amount of emotional space it causes us to take up in our loved ones' lives. Take *Welcome to Me*, a 2014 indie film about Alice Klieg (Kristen Wiig), a woman with BPD who wins the lottery and launches her own daytime *Oprah*-esque talk show. When I learned of the film, I was as excited as I was ahead of the Yale keynote. There was finally an irreverent comedy that didn't pair the disorder with institutionalization, violence, or criminality.

Klieg's daytime television show is a surprise hit in the ratings likely due to what her mother deems her emotional exhibitionism, and it leads Klieg to alienate and neglect her best friend, Gina Selway (Linda Cardellini). An accident on set where Alice "nearly burns her tits off" sets off her mental deterioration. It takes the form of an emotionally devastating montage of dogs getting neutered, a series of lawsuits brought forward by people she's defamed on her show, a nude walk through the casino she's living in, and an eventual hospitalization. Selway delivers a teary speech when she finally visits Klieg in the hospital. "You're a terrible friend," she tells Klieg. "You only care about your own pain. I'm sorry you hurt so bad, but that doesn't mean other people aren't vulnerable or sensitive and just because you've made a career out of it doesn't mean other people don't have feelings." Klieg melts into a puddle of tears. "You don't get to fucking cry right now," Selway says. "I am crying right now." *Welcome to Me* frames BPD as a bigger burden to support networks than it is for the sufferer.

So how can the media industry do a better job of representing BPD to the masses? Simple. Let people with the disorder inform or create characters with BPD. In the rare case when this happens, like in *Ida's Diary*, a 2014 documentary account of living with BPD, we see people with the disorder strive instead of simply struggle. We watch Ida, a woman who admits she's afraid of living as much as she's afraid of dying, climb Norway's highest mountain. She smiles shyly at the camera when she reaches its peak. We see her highs as well as her lows. We see her humanity. And Pete Davidson is exploring what life with the disorder looks like for men in his semi-autobiographical film *King of Staten Island* and television series *Bupkis*. Of course, common to all these depictions is the centring of whiteness. We need an array of experiences represented in media depictions of the disorder that unpack how factors like systemic racism influence the course and treatment of living with BPD—experiences that I or any of the characters in this essay can't embody.

✳

In her closing statement to the jury, Vasquez reminded them that she had kept her promise of presenting Heard as a "deeply troubled person" who had a dreadful impact on Depp's life due to her alleged personality disorders. "[Heard is] desperate for attention and approval. And in her relationship with Mr. Depp, she was violent, she was abusive, and she was cruel . . . Ms. Heard suffers from borderline personality disorder and histrionic personality disorder. These are disorders that are characterized by anger, sometimes uncontrollable and explosive anger, and a powerful and sometimes desperate need for attention, acceptance, and approval. Fear of abandonment is the deepest fear. A person with these disorders will suffer from dramatically fluctuating moods and can sometimes be violent and aggressive."

What happens between two people behind closed doors is always going to be up for debate, especially if one of those people has BPD. Legally, things never went as far for me as they did for Heard. But how much more damaged and invalidated would I have felt if I had to defend my accusations and behaviours on a public stage? Would my allegations be received as the sick ramblings of a broken mind? Based on how women who acted like me have been treated in the media, I suspect I would be more likely to end up cast as an untrustworthy monster than a sick person who had been victimized. In this way, I'm lucky. I can hold onto my truth in the absence of the spotlight's harsh glare.

The ruling on the Depp-Heard defamation case was presented on June 1, 2022. The Virginia jury found that Heard had defamed Depp through her op-ed. They awarded him $10 million in compensatory damages and $5 million in punitive damages (though this was later reduced to $350,000 due to a limit prescribed by state law). Heard, who had countersued Depp for $100 million for statements Depp's lawyer Adam Waldman made, was awarded $2 million in compensatory damages and no punitive damages. The two later settled, which involved a $1-million payment to Depp.

At the time of writing, Depp is on a comeback tour. He's performed with Jeff Beck, appeared in Rihanna's *Savage x Fenty Vol. 4* fashion show, and was feted at Cannes for his turn in *Jeanne du Barry*, a French film with Depp in the role of King Louis xv. Meanwhile, Heard left the U.S. to live quietly with her daughter in Europe.

There will never be a broad reckoning on the nature of the abuse I believe I was a victim of in childhood. The closest I came was a phone call during the Depp-Heard trial. My granny asked me to catalogue the precise forms my punishments took, how often it happened, and what it felt like while I was experiencing it. It was the closest I felt she ever came to recognizing the abuse I experienced in my childhood. But I knew it would only take one conversation between my granny and my stepdad to undo the emotional labour of that phone call. Violence is tempting to overlook or minimize. Especially when it happens to someone who is considered unreliable.

Unlike me, Heard isn't so lucky. Her case was already decided by both a literal court and the court of public opinion despite an open letter signed by over 130 organizations and individuals in support of her experience. The spotlight set Heard aflame. It made her op-ed more relevant than when it was initially published.

On paper, Depp won the trial. But Heard isn't the real loser here. The real losers are the people with BPD who will think twice about speaking about our experiences or reaching out for help if we're the victim of a crime.

COMPANION PLANTS

I. SPROUT

My mother wasn't the type to have a boisterous group of friends she regularly met for dinner. She didn't go out once a week to shoot darts like my stepdad did. She didn't sit on the PTA. In the rare moments she wasn't working to support the family, running after me or my brother, or cleaning up after the pets, she liked to garden. She made gardens any place we lived long enough to plant them.

I remember spraying arcs of refracted water streams on tidy rows of petunias in the backyard of our first townhouse. I watched sadly when she cleared out a jungle of prickly rose bushes that gave our Bowmanville backyard a witchy, haunted look. She rounded the edges of garden beds at our semi-detached house in Uxbridge, shading her brow with her hand when she stopped to talk to our Baptist neighbour, whose children only knew hymns and songs from *VeggieTales*. The next house had a sliver of a yard that backed onto the town's water treatment plant—a solitary pumphouse sitting on an acre of fenced-in land, where my stepdad flung the dog's poops. She framed its borders with tulips, climbing beans, daffodils, and vine tomatoes all the same.

My mother had learned the pleasure of sowing a hope and watching it blossom into something real from her mother, who learned it from hers, all the way back to my great-great-grandmother, the medicine woman of the small Ukrainian village our family comes from. She had crushed leaves into poultices to heal her neighbours' rashes, brewed herbal teas to soothe sore throats, and used plant life like poppy seeds to relieve pain. (This medicinal herbal knowledge was mostly lost to our family over time and through the stunting nature of war and displacement.)

I didn't care for the dirt. It was my younger brother who loved to learn about plants. He squatted on his small haunches and watched my mother prod seeds beneath the soil. The sun created a golden halo in his blonde hair. Each spring, he was responsible for his own vine, but his beans never made it inside the house. He'd pop a bean into his little pink mouth as soon as one was fat and ripe, ecstatic to taste the fruits (or vegetables) of his labour.

I preferred to dig through my mother's jewellery box. She told me stories of who she had been before she became my mother while I stroked her pearls and strung her gold chains through my chubby fingers. She reminisced about admirers who had given her rings or necklaces—enough pieces that she had them melted down into something shiny and new. She had the type of beauty that inspired obsession. One of her exes became so enthralled he planted himself in the bushes by her home. Perhaps the most astute were determined to run dry the well of sorrow they sensed within her heart without realizing that everyone who tried had soaked themselves to the bone—the same depths I tried to distract her from when she shared tales of her beauty.

I matched my mother in sadness when I reached adulthood, but my looks didn't inspire infatuation. I was more likely to be the person looking in from the outside than the one admired like a blossom.

I caught a glimpse of M., the online editor, on the first day of my internship at an esteemed if occasionally overregarded magazine operated as a nonprofit. Coffee in hand, he hustled across the bright newsroom to retreat into the lamplit office he shared with another "propeller head," which is how the executive director referred to the guys responsible for Internet stuff. I liked his scruffy beard and the way his eyes twinkled. Then I noticed the shiny gold ring on the fourth finger of the hand that held his coffee. I poked the seed of attraction I felt for him deep into the murk of my subconscious.

Buried things cannot be ignored forever. Eventually, the ideal conditions will come along, the pod the secret lives inside of swells and bursts, and a tiny green leaf gains the energy it needs to poke its head from the soil.

II. SEEDLING

Fridays at the office were often boozy. At four in the afternoon, we ignored the emails pinging our BlackBerrys and gathered in a manager's office to drink whatever bottles were left over from fundraising events.

A few years after I was hired as a full-time event coordinator, three or four of us were gathered in M.'s office. M. played DJ on his computer. I sat on a well-worn IKEA loveseat next to the circulation director and sipped rum and Coke from a coffee-stained mug.

"You okay?" the circulation director asked M. "You seem kind of down."

M. was usually a wonderful storyteller, just like my mother. His normally passive face animated as if someone had flicked an internal switch to *on* when he started recounting a tale. His eyes would shine while he set a scene. His hands would meander like a painter dabbing bits of colour onto canvas before the whole artwork came together. He would pause to draw out the suspense of the climax, his audience listening with hands cradled beneath their chins and eyes as wide as coins. His punchlines were delivered flawlessly and always elicited the desired response.

But that day, M.'s words seemed to stick in his throat. He shrugged, pursed his lips, and tilted his head from side to side. "I'm getting divorced," he said finally.

We expressed our sympathies, and a silence settled over the room. I reflected on my false conviction that love could conquer all. I supposed it began with the Disney princess films my mother loaded into the VHS player on rainy days. Cartoon women with tiny waists and big chests had all their problems solved when a person with a penis showed up. It gave me the impression that unconditional love would alleviate my emotional problems.

In the house with the rounded flower beds, my bedroom window faced the sleepy street—the neighbourhood's main thoroughfare. I was able to pry out the window screen on warm nights and crawl onto the garage roof. Far enough from the city's light pollution, the stars watched me watch the road.

I used to wish that a passing car would slow and stop in front of our driveway. My biological father, a man I had never met, had served as an imaginary stand-in for the type of safe love I longed for. He would emerge from the vehicle's opening door, ready to spirit me into the night. We'd drive away from the household I never fit into, where I was taught to navigate moods like minefields, where it was more comfortable to dig a tunnel into a snowdrift and crawl into it with a good book than spend an afternoon trapped inside with my stepdad, where tears were more common than smiles, and where premature death would be welcome since it meant not having to face the long and lonely years ahead.

Two decades after those nights on my roof and five years after that afternoon in the office, I sat on the balcony's cement step outside the apartment I shared with M. while I vaped, a compromise since M. hated the smell of cigarettes. I watched a viral video of two houseplants raised in identical environments under similar conditions: each plant received an equal amount of light, water, and attention. But the attention came in different forms. The plant on the right side of the screen was praised and encouraged. The plant on the left was belittled and bullied. Both plants stretched from their pots. The well-loved plant grew tall and sturdy. It sprouted fresh frog-green leaves. The other plant grew dark. It withered and drooped; the plant's few leaves curled into angry fists.

I can't find the original clip I watched to confirm so this may be a hopeful figment of my imagination, but the bullied plant was praised after the experiment was over. Its leaves relaxed. Over a time-lapse, the colour returned to its skin. It started to look more like its nurtured peer.

III. VEGETATIVE

In grade school, I went through a phase in which I dotted the *I* in my name with a little heart on homework assignments. It was a nod to my intense devotion to the feeling and a question to those who saw it: "Won't you give me the validation that I need?" I pined for the sort of romantic love that would affirm my redeemability, anchor me through the storms of my emotions, and unearth strengths I wasn't even aware I had long before I had a face to attach to the feeling. Reality show contestants and D-list actresses from my favourite science fiction series were the focus of my early fantasies. I dreamed of a world where I was as pretty as my mother instead of a chubby girl with gaps between my crooked teeth and permanent dark circles that shadowed my eyes. In these intricate scenarios, my cast of lovers held me when I was scared, wiped tears from my cheeks with soft fingers, and told me I was the best thing that had happened to them all with the earnestness of an afternoon soap opera. I couldn't wait for bedtime or lengthy car rides so I could return to the protective world that lived behind my eyes.

My affections took on a similar obsessiveness when it came time to transplant my fantasies into reality. I was prone to intense entanglements with a half-life that faded fast. I'd learn later that these fervent attachments are common to people with BPD. People with the disorder often experience acute devotion to a single person (a friend, family member, or romantic partner) who influences their mood, identity, and self-worth. The focus of these intense relationships is known as the "favourite person," or FP, within the BPD community. People with the disorder idolize their FPs, rely on them for support, and feel like they can't function when that person isn't in their life. It's a heavy dependency thought to be the result of not receiving enough early validation from caregivers.

At first, M. and I kept our budding relationship secret. I didn't report to him, but he was a manager while I was still a lowly coordinator. The optics weren't great. We stayed subtle by communicating mostly through email during office hours. I always signed off with only my first initial, a habit I had picked up years earlier. It hinted at the space I was willing to take up in a relationship—almost none. My initial could have been a mistyped letter, easy to overlook, and hopefully small enough to be welcomed into an inbox or at least not immediately deleted from it. That M. and I shared the same initial gave me a little thrill. I could be indistinguishable from him.

People with BPD will adopt their FP's preferences or opinions to please them. M. and I had quite a bit in common but I accentuated the parts of myself I felt attracted him most, like my affinity for old-school hip-hop. I diminished the habits he disliked, like my fondness for recreational stimulants. It's the same strategy used by flowers: the hammer orchid resembles a female wasp to lure pollinating males; carrion flowers mimic the scent and appearance of rotting flesh to attract pollinators like flies and beetles. It was easier to believe that M. loved the parts of his personality that I mirrored back to him rather than any of my own qualities.

I had built up a tall and sturdy pedestal to place M. upon by the time our first summer together arrived. Like all favourite people, he could do no wrong in my eyes. I felt lucky to linger in his shadow and wanted to spend each waking moment in the refreshing curves of his silhouette.

"What time are you thinking of heading home?" he asked one blazing afternoon. We sat across from each other and shared a joint on his second-storey balcony, which was sheltered by an ancient maple tree.

"You want me to go?"

"Well," he said with a hint of regret in his voice. "It's not that I want you to go. It's just that I have to get some work done. And we have spent the last three days together . . ."

Later, I stayed quiet as we walked past colourful gardens, fat yellow bees drunk on nectar, and squirrels scaling up thick tree trunks on our way to the subway. I was devastated. I couldn't fathom why M. didn't want to neglect all of his responsibilities and other relationships to spend time with me. I would drop everything for him with unparalleled devotion. Of course, I didn't tell him any of this. I was afraid any expression of disappointment would drive him away.

We parted with a kiss. I couldn't still my bouncing knees or stop tearing at my ragged cuticles with my teeth as the subway car screamed toward Broadview station. Visions of bitter partings haunted me. By the end of the ride, I had convinced myself that M. was no better than the favourite people I had left in the past: the boyfriend from university who had refused to accompany me to my abortion when we got pregnant, the best friend from high school who disappeared into her first relationship, or the person my mother was before she married.

It's inherently precarious to worship at an FP's pedestal. The pillar crumbles with the passage of time. Minor transgressions create cracks of fear and doubt. People with BPD rely on an instinctual defence mechanism known as splitting or black-and-white thinking when these cracks occur. The strategy presents as a failure or difficulty to simultaneously hold opposing thoughts, beliefs, or feelings—like the idea that my partner could care about me and also need to spend time away from me. It means that a person with BPD views themselves and others as all good or all bad when triggered, which results in a cycle of overidealizing and devaluing. Splitting works by protecting the ego and reducing anxiety. Disappointment becomes less painful if I expect my loved ones to let me down. Goodbyes aren't as difficult once I've minimized a person's positive qualities. My perception creates my reality.

I have no control over when I split. But once I learned about the mechanism it was easier to identify when it was happening and live with the distortion or do the cognitive work required to overcome it. It was like having a trauma flashback. It was scary and disorienting to have the past eclipse the present, but the waking nightmare wasn't as distressing if I kept reminding myself that it wasn't real.

Ultimately, it was M. who gave me the confidence to stand by my name. My full name. We were waiting to board a flight to Bermuda a few months after our first summer together. Nearby, children shrieked, barely discernable warbled flight announcements crackled overhead, and cash registers chimed relentlessly. My laptop was open on my lap, my face aglow, my brow wrinkled in frustration.

"I need to file this piece before we go," I said to M., who had been trying to read a magazine. "And I have no idea how to fucking finish it."

I was firmly entrenched in the fundraising side of nonprofit publishing and had even found a new job as an event manager, but I still wanted to be a writer. I had tiptoed back into writing simple Q & As in my off-hours after the brain fog from a particularly strong course of antipsychotics had cleared. That's what the assignment had started out as. And then the editor-in-chief decided that the format was unfashionable—better it become an opinion piece. Strong opinions defied my nature, but I wanted the byline. I agonized over each word the way many fledgling writers do, whined when it was nearly reassigned, and failed to keep my patience when it was passed from editor to editor before it landed in the hands of a new hire.

"Mention that to the editor," he said. "That's what they're there for."

"Are you kidding me? She introduced spelling errors in my last draft. I don't trust her to make my words read well. Please, I need your help. Otherwise, I'm just going to pull the whole thing."

M. took my laptop. He tucked the bottom of his beard into the neck of his shirt the way he always did when he was editing. "This reads better than you think it does," he said. He scrolled through the document, his crooked pinkie finger, broken from basketball, unattended and poorly healed, hovered over the trackpad. His hands danced across the keyboard. "How about this?" he asked and passed back the computer.

He had added two sentences to the bottom of the page, two sentences that tied together everything that I was trying to say. "Yeah, okay," I said. "Thank you." I emailed the draft to the editor.

Our flight was called to board just as I snapped the lid of my computer shut. Those two sentences survived the editing process and can still be found in the article today. The first opinion piece I published under my full name.

IV. BUDDING

A gentle breeze blew through the barren branches that quivered above me. I plunged my pitchfork deep into black earth tangled with roots and ragged weed fabric that the landlord had installed a decade ago and promptly abandoned. I paused to wipe the film of sweat that had formed across my brow with the sleeve of one of M.'s lumberjack coats before I turned the soil over. Dirt was packed beneath my fingernails. An unseen woodpecker tapped out a series of notes that soundtracked my slow progress in readying the garden for planting.

I had time to tackle the ignored plot of land that our downstairs neighbours, who had seen me milling aimlessly around the block, suggested I take over.

A few months after our trip to Bermuda, I had woken up with a panic so powerful it filled the inside of my head with the sound of screaming. Outpatient counselling did nothing to silence it. M. walked me to the hospital during a rainstorm. He kept shifting our tiny shared umbrella to try to cover both of us, but we arrived at the emergency room soaked and shivering. I resigned myself to inpatient psychiatric care for the second time. Since M. and I no longer worked together, I had assumed that once I was securely locked behind ward doors in a dry hospital gown, he'd vanish into the city's countless faces. My illness was too much to ask a partner to cope with. But he kept showing up to visiting hours with books, caffeinated coffee, and writing utensils—psych ward essentials. I couldn't return to full-time work when I was discharged. I lived off freelance gigs, evening usher jobs, and the meagre savings I'd banked until it became clear I wouldn't be able to afford my apartment in Greektown for much longer. M. asked me to move in with him slowly and cautiously. The way a person might invite a stray animal into their home.

With wide swaths of afternoon unoccupied, I had to find a project to wash away the hours. Some might believe people who cannot work as a result of mental illness are lazy or weak, but I wanted something to keep me busy. I had spent the winter tracing my dead grampa's roots to be closer to him in his absence and found a branch that stretched all the way back to the 1700s before census records dwindled. Spring had arrived while I was turned to the past. I needed something to ground me in the present. The nervous habits I'd acquired over time—nail-biting, moaning, and hyperextending my knees and elbows—didn't present when I'd pulled weeds on my walk home from grabbing a coffee one apathetic afternoon.

The act of creating sustainable terrain and nurturing a living thing takes patience, practice, and advice. I consulted with my mother on pruning groundcover conifers, the merits and drawbacks of using a jet-black mulch I had my eye on, and the difference between perennials and annuals. "If you can get the soil loosened and ready for planting, I can bring cuttings from my garden down on the bus," she said one night over the phone. Her voice carried hints of excitement that hadn't sparked between us in years. She advocated for planting vegetables—at least some herbs. I was adamant it should be a flower garden since the area doubled as a bathroom for neighbourhood cats. "Something bright and cheerful to look at," my granny agreed.

There was another reason I enjoyed the freedom found outside in the garden. A reason I didn't want to admit to myself. I was having trouble adjusting to cohabitation. Like a shelter dog, I wasn't necessarily housebroken. I approached everything from the side with a downward glance, anticipating a swat on the nose.

I don't remember if I knocked it off the couch, flung it from the bed when I tossed back the covers, or dropped it from the counter where I kept it balanced during my baths, but sometime after I moved in, I cracked M.'s iPad. A spiderweb of shattered glass scarred its corner. I brought the damaged device to him. Its face was cradled in my hands. Tears flowed down my cheeks.

"I'm so sorry." I explained what had happened. "I really can't afford to replace it right now. I understand if you'd like me to leave. I just need a few days to make arrangements."

M. chuckled sadly and wrapped his arms around me. I tensed in preparation for a final goodbye. "Of course you don't have to leave. It's just an object. No big deal," he said.

I travelled to Greece the summer before M. and I began dating. It was there I learned that the ancient Greeks had two concepts of time: χρόνος (chronos) and καιρός (kairos). Chronos is time as I always understood it—the chronological and quantitative march forward. Dawn fades to dusk, winter thaws into spring, and youthful skin sags and forms wrinkles. Kairos is more qualitative. Its nature is more permanent than chronos. It's an opportune moment or season—the only time when an action can occur. In an article published in *The Monist*, author John Smith identified two other concepts related to kairos: it's a time of crisis or conflict that calls for a decision, and it's a time when the opportunity to accomplish a purpose presents itself as a result of a problem that led to the crisis. Harvest time can be understood as kairos—the opportune moment to pluck a berry from a bush. Bone-white fruits turn carmine and call for a decision. Pick too early, and the berry will be tough and sour. Too late, and the berry will rot and ferment.

Trauma turns time cyclical. The things that happened to me are always happening to me. A lip curling into a sneer, a note of irritation in a normally melodic voice, or an unanticipated flick of the wrist all present as the golden hour for violence or neglect. I read M.'s body language the way farmers look to the colour of the sky to predict the weather. But something was amiss with my internal emergency alarm. Kairos was always lurking like a long-suppressed memory ready to overwhelm my reality. The opportune moment for danger was always.

The divide between the proper time for rest or action crystallized more clearly in the garden than it did within the walls of our apartment. Inside, I couldn't tell when it was the best time to use our shared washroom so I held my pee and wound up with a bladder infection. Outside, the opportune time of day for watering the flowers my mother delivered was in the morning before the stifling heat of that particular summer made their leaves wilt. Inside, cleaning the house was a constant duty. An obligation I felt to compensate for my lack of financial stability. In the fresh air, I only plucked the heads of my zinnias to encourage a second bloom once they shrivelled and dried into faded wisps. My internal clock was healing.

I muttered to my blossoms in rudimentary Ukrainian all summer long, trying to channel the way my baba (great-grandmother in this context) used to bend over and converse with her plants, once cultivating a thriving peanut bush inside her apartment. I photographed green stalks blooming into pale-orange lilies, coral poppies, crimson dahlias, and pink lupins. I sent the photos to my granny and my mother as if to say, *I might not be able to take care of myself very well right now, but look at the beautiful displays I've managed to grow since I found the right environment.*

V. FLOWERING

I shuffled downstairs bleary-eyed. The gauzy morning sky filled the apartment with blue shadows while I put on the kettle and ground the hipster coffee beans M. preferred. A frustrated sigh parted my lips when I reached the sink to rinse out the coffee press. A mostly empty yogurt container sat in its silver mouth. It was soaking in milky white water and emanated a sour smell.

I hate yogurt. I always have. Its scent summoned memories of chaotic lunches at unlicensed daycares, peeing my pants during snack time in junior kindergarten, and gagging after being told I wasn't allowed to leave the table unless my bowl was empty.

On most mornings, I held my breath, blasted the container with water until floating white chunks ceased to crest its lip, knocked it on its side to empty the vessel, and delivered it to the recycling with a pair of kitchen tongs without saying a word. On this morning, I left the container where it sat.

This minuscule change in habit was seeded months earlier. A close friend had married in a sprawling multi-day wedding ceremony. Her father, a man with a small stature and a large grin, worked the reception like a mafia don. He shook hands with tuxedoed guests, nodded happily at his relatives, and inquired loudly over the music's bass about the quality of the buffet. Plates were scraped, drinks were drained, and I grew morose. Both of my grandfathers were dead. If I were to ever marry, there would be no father figure aglow with pride to walk me down the aisle, to elbow guests as if to say, *Look at my beautiful girl*. I belonged to no one but myself.

My depression deepened and magnified over the weekend. Panic layered on top of it. By Monday, I was barely able to muster the energy to leave my bed. I ended up, briefly, in emergency inpatient psychiatric care at CAMH instead of my office (I'd returned to managing events) before I was referred to outpatient services.

My therapist's office was lit with a geode lamp, filled with houseplants, and decorated with artwork from the people she'd helped— so different from the clinical corridor just beyond her door. She wore no makeup and kept her curly brown hair pushed back with a fabric headband I strongly suspected was hemp.

We talked about BPD. There was still some question as to whether that was the right read on my mental illness. That M. and I had been together for four years had given other professionals pause. A key feature of BPD is having tumultuous relationships or relationships that the *DSM* characterizes as "intense and unstable . . . often viewed in extremes of idealization and devaluation."

"I can relate to most of the symptoms," I told the occupational therapist. "Except for the anger. I don't really get angry. My brain flags the feeling as dangerous and sort of converts it to sadness instead."

She gave me a soft therapist's smile and said, "When someone tells me they can't get angry, what I really hear is they have a problem setting boundaries."

I frowned and blinked a few times while I processed her words. My perception of anger was all twisted faces, bared teeth, flying spittle, animal-like rage-filled eyes, violence, and pain. To be angry was to lose control. It also required a fearlessness and self-possession that I lacked. Anger, it seemed, was for other people far stronger and more confident than I was.

"What if anger isn't about losing control or hurting someone?" my therapist asked. "What if we reframe anger as a natural reaction to our boundaries being violated?"

We spent the next few sessions in her hospitable office chiselling away at my certainty that it was my obligation to accommodate every request a loved one made, that their comfort was undoubtedly a priority over mine. She helped me identify habits and behaviours that bothered me. We practised setting small and manageable boundaries.

The stairs creaked beneath M.'s footsteps. I watched him drain his coffee mug and exhaust his morning yawns. The yogurt container's presence hovered in my mind like a power saw's whine. I cleared my throat until he looked up from reading basketball updates on his phone.

"Can I talk to you about something?" I asked. My hands trembled. My heartbeat was so fierce it sounded like a jackhammer. I tried to sink deeper into the leather couch, to anchor my body in its cushions, but my trunk was numb. There was a blankness where the feeling of my pyjamas should have been.

M. jerked in the armchair that my cats had clawed up when he noticed my nervousness. His eyes shifted from blurred and dreamy to alert with a flash of concern. "Of course. Is everything okay?" "No, actually." My chest tightened until my airway felt like a pinhole. Tears stung in my eyes. I rocked back and forth and rubbed my palms across my thighs to spark a soothing sensation but felt nothing. "I really don't like it when you leave empty yogurt containers in the sink. I hate it, actually. They smell terrible, and I detest cleaning them. It's not a very nice way to start my morning."

I held my breath. My gaze was fixed on the scratched wood floor. I winced and waited for his reaction.

M.'s whispery laugh filled the living room. His face wasn't angry or irritated when I looked up. "No problem," he said. "I'll rinse them out before I go to bed. I didn't realize it bothered you so much."

I let out a steady stream of breath. My heart rate slowed and my hands settled.

Studies show that those with BPD have a lower probability of experiencing enduring romantic relationships and are more likely to encounter low satisfaction or distress within a partnership. However, well-functioning relationships can act as a protective factor for people with BPD, leading to mental health stabilization and a reduction of symptoms. It reminds me of companion planting, a gardening strategy that involves planting different species together for mutual benefits like pest control or crop yield.

My baba had explained the approach to me when I was a girl. I had trailed her across the parking lot of her Ukrainian retirement home in Scarborough (or Scarberia, as she liked to call it) to the small garden plot she was allowed to keep at the edge of the grounds. We crouched in the dirt next to tidy vegetable rows. She waved a wrinkled hand, already stiff with creeping arthritis, toward bunches of fluffy green leaves, which I mistook for dill, interspersed with a plant with long straight shoots. "Carrot and onion," she explained in her broken English. "They friends. They sit next to each other. They grow good together." I learned later that the smell of onions deters the carrot root fly and the carrots repel onion flies.

A companion complements its partner. Together, they create a more nourishing environment. A companion's steady guiding presence allows those who surround it to reach their fullest potential.

VI. RIPENING

As I write, I notice myself glancing at the ring on the fourth finger of my left hand every few seconds. It catches the light like dust motes drifting by the window.

It's a new addition to my hand. It sits on top of a tattoo celebrating my and M.'s fifth anniversary. Its diamond cluster perfectly obscures the Roman numeral for five. I had never imagined someone would love me for so long and so well. I had wanted a reminder of our relationship to look down on when I was wrinkled and alone, assuming we wouldn't marry due to my aversion to events and M.'s prior history with the institution. I sat in our bathroom, dipped a needle into India ink, and carefully poked the integer into my skin, wiping away the odd speck of blood or extra smear of blackness. It had felt important to do the tattoo myself; the fresh scar was an act of love I only wanted to share with M.

The engagement ring I wear is actually my third. The first was too loose, two sizes too big and slipped right from my bony finger onto the candlelit table at our local Lebanese haunt where M. proposed a few months after we'd marked eight years together. He had hoped to surreptitiously measure one of the rings I wore on my right hand, as my brother had done before he proposed to his longtime partner, but I never remove them.

I can never quite tell when something fits. Half of my clothes are too large, even the ones I begrudgingly tried on in cramped dressing rooms, my patience for shopping already spent. I don't have a good sense of myself so it takes me a long time to be certain something is the right fit. When we exchanged the first ring at the pampas-grass-filled jewellery shop, I walked out with a piece of bling that was still too big, spinning freely around my finger, its stones biting into my palm when I made a fist.

I wasn't born from love. My biological father didn't propose to my mother or even get close to giving her a bit of gold I'd admire later. I was just a confluence of mistakes—a drunken New Year's Eve party, fumbling limbs in what I assume was a darkened guest room, the snap of a condom breaking. I emerged into the world a few decisions and nine months later, the responsibility of a single parent. I used to believe that a person couldn't find love if they weren't born from it. That my personality was too disordered for it. That love was as rare as a diamond.

This conviction was reinforced when I was officially diagnosed with BPD. Theoretically, a person with the disorder shouldn't be capable of performing the care necessary to maintain a relationship. The disorder's very definition implies that people with it don't have the secure attachment styles, sense of identity, mentalization skills, or emotional balance necessary for coupled life. But statistics tell a different story. One study found between 30 and 45 per cent of people with BPD are involved in romantic partnerships. It's below the national marriage rate in Canada (which sat at around 59 per cent before the pandemic), but it's certainly not an impossibility nor is it rare.

Diamonds aren't really that rare either. In 2019, 142 million carats of diamonds were pulled from mines around the world. The perception of rarity was created by De Beers Consolidated Mines Ltd., a group of major investors who took control of the industry in the nineteenth century when diamonds were flooding the market. The group kept prices high by restricting how many diamonds were on offer at any given time, only releasing enough rough stones to satisfy the current demand. De Beers linked the diamond to love during the Great Depression. The group hired N.W. Ayer and Son to create a slogan that would compel people to buy diamonds when proposing. "A diamond is forever" became synonymous with engagements. By 1999, the stockpile of diamonds De Beers hadn't released into the market was valued at 5.2 billion dollars. In 2004, the group pled guilty to price fixing in a U.S. federal court. It seems diamonds are as common as dandelions.

We drove back to the jewellery store for a final time just as a storm settled over Toronto. The roads were pure white, no snow plows were in sight, and few drivers braved the blizzard. Still, the store was bustling with last-minute Christmas shoppers, confused guys poring over glass displays, and chic salespeople buzzing around with brisk efficiency. A salesperson confused us with another couple when we approached the counter. "I'm so glad you decided not to propose in the Bahamas," she told M. We exchanged puzzled glances. We had no upcoming travel plans. She realized her mistake, eventually.

Right before he proposed, M. said to me, "You told me recently that you never thought you would lead a normal life. That made me really sad because you of all people deserve a normal life."

I was smiling when I left the store that day. Not simply because I had committed to a wonderful man and had a perfectly sized ring to show off during the holidays, but because we had been mistaken for an ordinary couple. I had found normalcy.

MOTUS TEMPESTAS

"I'm having a lot of trouble feeling anything," I told my therapist during a midday session. "And I don't mean just my emotions. My body too. It feels like I'm watching myself from above, which makes it difficult to stay in the present. It's really frustrating."

My therapist nodded and told me it made a lot of sense. When under stress, a person with BPD can dissociate entirely, feeling disconnected from their body and the world around them. "But let's take a moment to acknowledge that the mechanism didn't develop out of nowhere," she said. "It's happening because at one point being dissociated helped you survive."

My therapist was right. I remembered living rough, drifting through the city like a fog, no more solid than a puff of steam from a sewer grate. The ubiquitous emptiness once served a protective purpose. It overpowered more uncomfortable emotions like fear, anxiety, or anger. It made an untenable situation bearable. I was able to navigate a long and lonely road a little easier when I cut off my emotions.

"Let's go inward and find that dissociated part," my therapist said.

I closed my eyes to focus internally. I saw a younger version of myself traipsing through the snowy tundra of suburban Richmond Hill, snow so high it went past the tops of my boots, got inside them, and froze my feet. I wanted to cry, but it wouldn't have changed anything. So, I had gone somewhere else in my mind, far away from my soggy boots and my aching shoulders. Far away from the emotional pain of being so alone.

"Can we catch that dissociated part up to your present circumstances? Let it know you're in a position now where that dissociation no longer serves you," my therapist said.

I tried to show that part of me that I was no longer a struggling teenager. I was an adult with a supportive partner far away in time from housing insecurity and the circumstances that led to it. The part seemed to hear what I was saying, but my dissociation didn't fade immediately. My therapist recommended that I supplement checking in with that part with physical sensations that would ground me. I was advised to stand barefoot on the grass for at least five minutes each day and really focus on feeling the earth beneath me.

There are few creatures more fundamentally misunderstood than the individual with borderline personality disorder. People with BPD are often referred to as emotional "storms." And what are storms but nature at its most sublime? Much of the behaviour that is often seen as incomprehensible to the average person becomes understandable, even rational, when considering the person with BPD's perspective—that the world is a dangerous and frightening place and one needs to adapt accordingly.

Human habits reflect predispositions that helped our ancestors survive, reproduce, and find success in a range of settings. Social conduct is motivated, in part, by instinct. Our behaviours are shaped by the demands of our environment. When viewed through the lens of evolutionary psychiatry, a person with BPD's abnormal behaviour becomes a stable adaptive strategy designed to suit a specific environment. It's only maladaptive when it persists outside the conditions it was intended for. When BPD is framed as an extreme adaptation rather than a deficient deviation from the norm, how others relate to people with the disorder (and how people with BPD see ourselves) changes for the better. Stigma could become less prevalent if our conduct is viewed as a strategy that served us in earlier environments.

It's estimated that BPD occurs in 1 to 2 per cent of the human population. This means there are somewhere between 80 and 160 million people with BPD living in the wild at any given time. That there are so many people living with BPD indicates that the behavioural variation must serve a necessary function. Otherwise, natural selection wouldn't allow it to persist.

Evolutionary psychiatry hinges on the belief that human behaviours reflect physical and psychological predispositions that helped our ancestors survive and reproduce, but how can suicide—the voluntary end to life—be considered an adaptive behaviour? The answer can be found in the animal kingdom.

In Southeast Asia, there's a small but enormous-eyed creature with elongated fingers, which help it cuddle close to the tree branches it sits in. The tarsier. Tarsiers are carnivorous mammals whose soft velvety fur and tiny size (around four inches tall) attract hordes of tourists to see those kept in captivity or living in sanctuaries. These shy animals have amazing hearing and prefer quiet settings and limited contact with humans. When stressed by loud surroundings, flashing cameras, or unwanted touch, or when placed into cages— only half of all wild tarsiers survive in captivity—the vulnerable primate bashes its head against a hard surface until it dies.

Tarsiers have never successfully mated while in captivity. Perhaps they fatally harm themselves not just out of extreme pain or as a way to escape torturous surroundings but also for an evolutionary reason. Natural selection tends to favour processes that result in reproduction. If a creature can't or won't successfully reproduce due to its circumstances, it's apt to be selected out of a population. The suicidal tarsiers could simply be beating nature to the punch.

Like the tarsier, people with BPD have extreme responses to untenable environments. People with the disorder are predisposed to suicidal or self-harming actions. Like a parrot that pulls out its feathers when unhappy, people with BPD have physical reactions to distress that can become fatal if sufficiently severe. We can find somatic pain a welcome distraction from all-consuming emotions. Or from the pervasive emptiness people with the disorder experience.

Many people with BPD carry caches of scars hidden on their bodies. Thick white marks carved by kitchen knives, or burned into the fleshy part of the leg just above the ankle, or a decades-old collage of lighter burns shaped like a smile on the upper arm, or minuscule bald spots where scar tissue prevents hair from growing. (If observed, these scars should not be remarked upon unless the person with BPD broaches the subject first.) According to a 2014 *Frontiers in Behavioural Neuroscience* article, self-harm "may be 'adaptive' insofar as it operates as an anti-dissociation mechanism that reaffirms an individual's desire to feel . . . [and provides relief from] negative emotions."

Self-injury and suicidal behaviour could be tied to people with BPD's trouble regulating anger. We might lose our temper frequently. The strength of our rage can clash with the facts of a situation. When a child is raised in a setting where their emotions aren't validated, their feelings are minimized or criticized by their caregiver, or their emotional experience is eclipsed by their caregiver's, they're likely to learn that strong emotional expressions are the only way to get attention from the people around them. Unfortunately, this belief can persist into adulthood if the person with BPD hasn't learned how to set boundaries and develop healthy communication styles.

As a result of self-harm and suicide attempts, people with BPD are often found in inpatient or outpatient care. Considered "high utilizers" of health care systems, which is one reason we're not particularly popular with those who treat us, people with BPD are most likely to be found in these settings following or during a crisis. A psychotic experience is one of the most common crises that leads a person with BPD to emergency care. Psychotic experiences happen when people lose contact with reality. They see or hear things that aren't there (hallucinations) or believe things that aren't true (delusions).

Psychosis encompasses a broad spectrum of symptoms and experiences. Ahead of my first hospitalization, red iridescent orbs floated across my field of vision, obscuring my grandparents' comforting faces. Barely audible whispers seemed to call my name incessantly and stole my ability to sleep. I was frightened. I saw every staircase, every sharp edge, every medicine cabinet and kitchen drawer as a sneering dare to self-destruct. Terror-struck and aware I was hallucinating, where else was I meant to turn for help but the hospital?

When I was hospitalized, I sat in my assigned room in the ward's locked unit, on my bed that was bolted to the floor, a chill blowing across my bare legs. Alone, dressed only in socks and the two gowns I was given when I was admitted, I scanned the room for a way out. The grey flecked floor tiles and the cement walls seemed to wink at me. "We're very strong," they whispered. "What if you smacked your head against us over and over until your skull cracked like an egg and all your pain poured out?"

Like tarsiers, people with BPD do best in environments that are supportive of their needs and sensitivities. Suicide or self-injury might be an extreme adaptive response to agonizing and prolonged circumstances that cause a person with the disorder immense pain.

Non-fatal suicidal behaviour serves a vital purpose if it connects a person with BPD with professionals who can help us develop the skills we lack and replace habits that no longer serve us. It can also indicate to professionals when more care is necessary; however, a focus on minimizing exposure to traumatic settings is crucial.

Some experts believe that people with BPD should only be hospital-ized when their personal safety is at risk. And, even then, only for brief periods of time.

Tarsiers aren't the only creature that engages in self-destruc-tive behaviour. In South America, there's a species of bee willing to sacrifice its life in the name of protecting its nest. The *Trigona hya-linata* is a non-stinging bee that uses its ten teeth to defend against attackers. In an experiment conducted by the University of Sussex, researchers gave the bees a choice: stop biting and survive or con-tinue fighting but suffer lethal damage. They gripped attacking bees' wings with forceps and began to pull. The bees would be able to save their wings if they loosened their bites. Yet 83 per cent of *Trigona hyalinata* bees kept biting until their wings separated from the joint, rendering them flightless and unable to return to their nest—essentially sacrificing their lives to protect their col-ony. Without a colony, a bee has nothing.

Mother octopuses also engage in deadly behaviours. In the days after the cephalopod births her only clutch of eggs, she frets over her unborn, stringing each egg into strands and cementing the strands to the walls of her den. The mother blows water bubbles over the eggs to keep them oxygenated. She only eats if an unlikely prey animal, like a crab, wanders close to her grasp. A few days later, she stops eating entirely. Her skin loses colour and she wastes away. In captivity, female octopuses have been known to tear off their own skin, eat the tips of their tentacles, and bang into the walls of their enclosures. In the wild, a dying mother octopus might scar her skin with gravel along the sea floor or use her suckers to create self-inflicted lesions. By the time her eggs hatch, the mother is dead or on death's doorstep. It's hypothesized that this process may occur to prevent overpopulation or to protect the octopus's young from cannibalism.

One evolutionary explanation for suicide and suicidal behaviours was developed by Denys deCatanzaro, a professor emeritus at McMaster University. He proposed that the likelihood of self-destructive behaviours hinges on two factors: an individual's reproductive value and how much of a burden they feel they place on their relatives. His theory was based on W.D. Hamilton's kin selection proposition, which hypothesizes that self-sacrifice—like the type seen in the *Trigona hyalinata* bees—may support the survival of kin even at a cost to the organism's own life. In the case of the mother octopus, a creature that only reproduces once, her self-destruction ensures her hatchlings have the resources they need to thrive.

Creatures could be more prone to suicide and self-harm because of physiological differences. In a recent study, scientists surgically removed the gland responsible for the reproductive behaviour in female octopuses, including death. The animals abandoned their egg clutches and began eating again, doubling their lifespans. Researchers also discovered that one of the molecules responsible for self-harming conduct in octopuses is present in humans. Elevated levels of 7-dehydrocholesterol, or 7-DHC, in humans are linked with Smith-Lemli-Opitz syndrome, a rare disease in which half of all sufferers engage in self-injurious behaviour.

In two separate studies, researchers found people with BPD had structural brain abnormalities. One study compared the brains of people with the disorder who attempted suicide in highly lethal manners to those who had survived less lethal attempts. Researchers found less grey matter in the brains of those who made more harmful attempts. In the other study, there was less grey matter found in multiple areas of the brain when those with BPD were compared to healthy controls, which suggests there could be specific neural circuits responsible for suicidal behaviour. Alternately, early experiences might shape the brain to develop in a way that facilitates self-destruction in extreme conditions. Childhood adversity can impede the brain's ability to regulate emotions and impulses.

Shame is one of the emotions thought to be strongly linked to suicide and self-injury in people with BPD. Some researchers even think of BPD as a chronic shame response—the feeling that we'll never be good enough. In early research on suicidality, American social psychologist Roy Baumeister proposed that suicide may be motivated by the permanent escape it provides to people who are painfully aware of their shameful qualities, feel inadequately prepared to change these attributes, and experience guilt around letting their loved ones down. This aligns with deCatanzaro's evolutionary explanation for suicide. People with BPD could be prone to self-destruct because they feel they place too heavy a burden on their loved ones. And a person with the disorder without a support network feels like they're nothing.

I have known what it's like to feel like a burden. Early on in my relationship with M., he wanted to calm himself down during an argument by going for a walk. Wrecked by the emotional turmoil and anxiety I had caused him and terrified by the threat of abandonment, I impulsively took the staircase banister in both hands. I bashed my head against it repeatedly. My partner, horrified, turned to see a smear of red on the handrail's white paint. Warm blood pooled on my head. It dripped down my face, following the path my tears took, and congealed into a sticky mess beneath my chin. When the emergency medical technicians arrived, one stopped dead in his tracks. "Jesus," he said when he saw me sitting in the stairway, my green eyes shining through my blood-drenched face.

My act might be seen by conventional psychiatry as manipulative—seemingly meant to prevent abandonment. But there's an evolutionary purpose for this fear. Historically, children who survived into adulthood were the ones who stayed close to and were dependent upon their caregivers for protection and resources.

But what if something deeper was at play than simply delaying my partner's exit or staying physically close to him? What if I saw the ways my instinctive responses harmed the person I loved most and, devastated by this realization, impulsively tried to self-destruct to save him some long-term grief? The explanation for my behaviour becomes harder to disparage when it's viewed through evolutionary psychology.

We don't know that animals are capable of the conscious intent necessary to die by suicide as humans understand the concept. Self-destructive behaviours in animals could be deeply instinctual strategies nearly impossible to overcome. But what if suicidality in people with BPD isn't so different? What if it's an instinctive biological response to untenable environments, extreme discomfort, or protect one's kin?

✳

Most people with BPD live fast lives. Those with the disorder have a life expectancy nearly twenty years shorter than the average human lifespan.

This is the same life expectancy found in people with significant trauma. From 1995 to 1997, Kaiser Permanente, an American health organization, investigated the impact of abuse, neglect, parental drug use, violence, and divorce on a child's health in the adverse childhood experiences (ACE) study. A child scored an ACE point for each traumatic experience they were exposed to, up to a maximum of ten. The more ACE points a person has, the worse their long-term physical and mental health are likely to be. That BPD is strongly associated with childhood trauma cannot be overlooked.

Like people with high ACE scores, people with BPD are apt to have physical health problems. People with the disorder are more likely to struggle with obesity, live a sedentary lifestyle, and be at increased risk for cardiovascular diseases. Eating disorders are common. Just as a high ACE count can be a predictor of poor sexual health, so can impulsivity in BPD.

We need only to follow my adolescence to see how these health problems can manifest and compound. My eating disorder began when I was a teenager, staring at the pale and puckered ring of fat around my belly in the mirror. I found my mother's laxatives in the medicine cabinet. I supplemented these with a few fingers down my throat until my impulsivity waned and it seemed easier and more rewarding to restrict my calories, adding up the day's intake onto a folded square of paper I kept tucked in my jeans pocket. I liked the emotional peace and sense of control this behaviour brought on when so much of my life seemed out of my hands.

When I learned that cigarettes are appetite suppressants, I may have pilfered the odd smoke from my mom's pack of Du Maurier Extra Lights. One study found that 78 per cent of adults with BPD develop an addiction at some point in their lives. After I developed my own, I found myself welcome in the "tough" crowd, the clique that offered the most protection, or so I believed based on the comportment I saw modelled by my Hells Angels–loving stepfather. It was a socialization strategy that persisted when I moved to a new town, where the cool kids didn't just smoke cigarettes and weed but railed lines of coke while they watched *Fear and Loathing in Las Vegas* or took the bus to dance at raves in downtown Toronto, pupils black and round as a solar eclipse. I learned to like the drugs because, for a few hours, my intense emotions were warranted. I could pretend to be just like everyone else.

I found myself spending most of my time in my grandmother's darkened spare bedroom the summer before I started university, nestled in a cloud of comforters and pillows, too exhausted to deal with apartment hunting or applying for student loans—a departure from my inclination to be organized. I thought I was sleeping to avoid the sharp pains on the right side of my belly, to conserve energy since I had no appetite, and to rest my aching joints. When I saw a doctor for the first time in years, I learned I had hepatitis A. A German study found BPD is associated with increased rates of HIV and hepatitis.

The medication I've been prescribed to deal with my symptoms, particularly antipsychotics, added to my body's metabolic burden. Side effects listed in the leaflets packaged with my meds include unusual bleeding, constant headaches, insomnia, increased suicidal thoughts and behaviours, lack of muscle control, confusion, tremors or tardive dyskinesia, substance dependence, memory loss, emotional blunting, withdrawal, seizures, aggression, hallucinations, irregular periods, high rates of infection, blood clots, weight gain, kidney problems, unwanted breast milk, and glaucoma. And then there are my own suicide attempts. Teenaged overdoses on over-the-counter medication like Tylenol, which can cause acute liver injury.

A person with BPD's suspicious nature can also interfere with physical health. We frequently struggle with paranoia, particularly about others' motives or intentions.

I recently refused to schedule an appointment for a Pap test with a new doctor. "He's been my doctor for a year and a half and we've never met. He didn't even call to introduce himself after he took over my old doctor's practice," I explained to my granny over the phone one morning. "And the first thing he wants to see is my vagina? I'm not comfortable with that."

"That sounds pretty fishy to me too," my grandmother said, because I had to learn my paranoia from someone. And that behaviour has kept generations of women in my family safe.

There are times when survival relies on quick responses. In environments that are chronically traumatizing, the inclination to live hard serves both people with BPD and those with a history of early adversity as it allows them to endure unusual situations. If a person with the disorder or a traumatized person subconsciously determines that the resources that we need to thrive are scarce—and these resources can be physical, emotional, or otherwise—we're apt to adopt a faster-paced life strategy. Faster-paced life strategies are typically associated with heightened threat sensitivity, low tolerance of frustration, poor executive control, neuroticism, low levels of consientiousness, agreeableness, harm avoidance, risk proneness, unstable interpersonal relationships, opportunism, heightened impulsivity, and novelty-seeking—behaviours that read similarly to the symptoms of BPD. It's a cruel twist of fate that the strategies that once protected us could now destroy us.

But a person with BPD doesn't need research studies to tell them this. It exhausts us to feel emotions so intensely. Like meteors, we burn bright but fade fast.

In the wild, many animals or plants like the carrion flower, which imitates the scent of rotting flesh to attract pollinators, use mimicry as an aggressive or defensive survival strategy. Mimicry can protect a species from predators, lure prey, or allow it to infiltrate optimal environments without being found out.

The rove beetle, for example, takes advantage of others' homes to meet its needs. The beetles used to enter ant or termite colonies to find prey. Over time, the beetles evolved to smell and look like ants. They infiltrated insect colonies and lived among them. In the safety of an ant colony, there is plenty of food (and ants) for the rove beetle to eat. Though they were once solitary creatures, these beetles adapted to become social insects.

People with BPD are also known to use mimicry, or mirroring, as an adaptive strategy. We experience rapid changes in self-identity and self-image. We can see ourselves as a generally good person one moment, only to feel evil the next. Occasionally, we might feel as if we don't exist at all. This fractured sense of self leads to shifting goals, values, career paths, and relationships. Similar to the chameleon, the person with BPD can alter their identity to camouflage in uncertain terrain and to socially signal to others. Often learned in childhood, this fluidity is key in unstable environments where survival and receiving aid are dependent on an ability to adapt to the unpredictable moods of caregivers.

Many humans subconsciously mirror others to fortify social networks and build a sense of belonging, but numerous studies have found that people with BPD engage in stronger behavioural mirroring compared to healthy participants. Some of the processes involved in mimicry are altered in people with BPD. In one study, people with BPD showed increased automatic mimicry of negative social signals—angry, sad, and disgusted facial expressions—and a reduced response to positive social cues. This might indicate that people with BPD are more likely to respond to negativity, which could account for some of the difficulties people with the disorder experience in interpersonal relationships. When a person grows up in an environment rife with negative social cues, they become accustomed to the behaviour. They look for it in others and use its presence as a warning sign.

I have frequently relied on mimicry to meet my needs. As a preteen, I spent nearly every weekend away from home sleeping over at friends' houses. One friend's father joked he should build another bedroom onto the house just for me since I stayed over so often. I winced and laughed nervously, part of me wishing I could tell the pleasant man who had an unending supply of dad jokes that I'd like nothing more than to join his safe and mild household and spend my evenings playing video games with his daughter or lounging in the solarium with his welcoming wife. In a different house, one my parents derisively referred to as "the yuppie house," I luxuriated in the routine of overhauling a century home, steaming and stripping off long sheets of gaudy wallpaper while listening to music on a candy-coloured iMac. My efforts were rewarded with a gift card to my favourite clothing store, American Eagle, a brand my parents couldn't afford. This behaviour was only reinforced when I was living rough, infiltrating other families' homes to find shelter like the rove beetle.

Some mimics are harmless creatures that take on the appearance of more dangerous critters in hopes they will be left alone. The coral snake and the scarlet kingsnake both have red, black, and yellow bands. The coral snake is extremely venomous. The scarlet kingsnake is harmless. The scarlet kingsnake copies the coral snake's markings to deter predators who mistake it for its more poisonous look-alike. Interestingly, this mimicry seems to persist even in areas where the coral snake no longer lives. In North Carolina, coral snakes haven't been seen since the 1960s; researchers assumed that the scarlet kingsnakes there would have evolved to look less like the missing coral snake. However, scarlet kingsnakes that were analyzed in the early aughts tended to look more like coral snakes than their ancestors from the 1970s. The research team hypothesized that when coral snakes started to decline, those that looked most like the venomous snakes were more likely to survive, hence the quick evolutionary adaptation.

My septum piercing was a defensive mimicry strategy. Before the piercing experienced a revival and could be found poked into the noses of pop stars and every other hipster, I befriended a girl at my high school with the rare piercing. I liked that the girl's jewellery, a metal horseshoe with two balls on each heel, could be flipped up into her nose. It disappeared in settings where it wasn't appropriate to look like a raging bull. But it also made her look intimidating. I was a country kid new to comprehensive local bus routes that could ferry teenagers to the city. I hoped a bullring would disguise my naïveté and deter predators willing to take advantage of my innocence—the strategy the scarlet kingsnake uses. I smiled whenever I heard "You'd be so pretty without that thing in your nose" or "That bullring is pretty scary." My mimicry was working.

The katydid is an insect that uses both aggressive mimicry (like the rove beetle) and defensive mimicry (like the scarlet kingsnake). These green bugs resemble plant life and are easily mistaken for the leaves that make up their environment, an adaptation that makes them harder for predators to find and eat. The spotted predatory katydid, or the *Chlorobalius*, lures in male cicadas for a tasty snack by imitating the female cicada's song, similar to the sirens from Homer's *Odyssey*, who use their heavenly voices to entice men to their end.

Mimicry has protected me when I've wandered into questionable circumstances. In 2019, I took a trip to the Bahamas to visit my grandmother. Used to relying upon the resources of others, I found myself drawn onto a yacht occupied by John McAfee, founder of the virus protection software everyone used in the nineties, Internet troll, and alleged rapist and murderer who died in 2021. I entered the cabin—unsure if it was from an urge to find weed or to be close to wealth, notoriety, and hence opportunity—to find cigarette butts floating in glasses of red wine, puddles of dog piss from the four beasts McAfee kept aboard for protection, and smudges of white residue on a glass table. McAfee was hosting a live stream for one of his presidential runs. A big Bahamian man with a warm welcoming smile sat next to him cradling an AK-47. The British fellow who'd invited me onto the yacht donned a mask of McAfee's face and passed me a lit joint and my own McAfee mask. I took both and put on the mask. I didn't want to be McAfee, but I was keenly aware I was the only woman on the boat. I'd be safer if I could be mistaken for one of the guys, like a katydid confused with a leaf. I hit the joint. Surrounded by real and fake McAfees, my head spun from the strong weed. I passed the spliff to the large fellow with the gun. I stayed on the yacht until the joint was spent, doing my best to blend into the scratched and drooled-on leather sectional. McAfee started to tell a story about a Thai stripper he knew who could squeeze a watermelon out of her vagina. I slipped out to the deck to "get some air" and clambered onto the wooden pier, my pace accelerating with each step away from the boat. I had what I needed from the encounter.

A person with BPD engages in resource exploitation (interpersonal or material) subconsciously, on instinct, based on predictions influenced by our early experiences. People who grow up in emotionally dangerous or unstable situations are inclined to see necessities like secure and trusting relationships as scarce or unpredictable. This scarcity compels people with BPD into a strategy of immediate resource acquisition, which is facilitated by an increased aptitude for mimicry.

✳

Faster paced life strategies affect how living things form relationships and reproduce. Life history theory predicts that creatures raised in environments where parental support is limited are more likely to engage in risky sexual behaviour and form short-term relationships when they reach maturity.

Look at the songbird. The songbirds have faster life histories than most other avian species. In a 2019 study, researchers found more promiscuous species had less male parental care during the nesting cycle, more short-term pairings, and more migratory behaviour. The study demonstrated the relationship between mating and the songbird's life pace. Tropical songbirds, typically slower-paced creatures, had more resources than their temperate counterparts and as a result produced fewer chicks, investing more into each individual, which led to a lower mortality rate. Temperate songbirds that led a faster life had fewer resources available and higher mortality rates. They adapted by producing a greater number of low-quality offspring.

Just as the person with BPD's life expectancy is influenced by a faster-paced life strategy, so is their sexual expression and reproduction. People with the disorder frequently act on impulse, especially when upset. Impulsive behaviours can include reckless spending, substance use, engaging in risky sex, dangerous driving, or binge eating.

Impulsiveness can be a useful skill in highly competitive settings, including environments where love and support are scarce. It allows the person with BPD to obtain aid from our habitat through quick reactions. But outside these environments, impulsivity can be damaging.

People with BPD tend to engage in sex earlier and have more sexual partners than their non-borderline peers. Additionally, women with the disorder are more likely to experience sexual coercion, intimate partner violence, and date rape. Although women with BPD change partners more often and reproduce less than other women, our relationship history may lead to a strategy that allows us to minimize our exposure to potentially dangerous partners while still engaging in reproduction or sexual expression. Impulsivity doesn't just affect a person with BPD's sexuality. It affects their relationships with others. These relationships often include a polarity of idealizing and devaluing behaviour. According to a 2009 *Medical Hypotheses* article, "Relationships with early caregivers decisively influences the way adults maintain relations afterwards . . . Having a negative emotional experience with caregivers during childhood precipitates the development of an abnormal mental model about relations." A child who receives inconsistent care or whose stage of development that allows them to see others as complex individuals is interrupted by trauma is predisposed to split between seeing a loved one as all good or all bad. This defence mechanism protects an individual from emotional conflict, perceived stress, and anxiety produced by contradictory perceptions of others. Splitting also serves an adaptive purpose. A 2004 *Theory and Psychology* article defines the mechanism (in normal populations) as "a universal cognitive process that acts to structure the world into predictable categories in order to facilitate perceptions of personal control and adaptive action."

When someone important in my life lets me down, I subconsciously fixate on their flaws and negate their redeeming attributes and the patient years they tended to our relationship. My perception of them shifts. I see them as "bad" or "dangerous," which makes it easier (and faster) to stop the relationship in its tracks. Splitting also offers emotional protection. If I expect a person to let me down, it won't be as painful when it happens.

A few weeks after I talked to my therapist about my struggles with dissociation, I was in a nearby park, barefoot, my toes pressing into the chilly spring grass. I had become more aware of my body in the intervening weeks. I had even presented my therapist with two sketches of myself. One was meant to depict how I felt before I worked on my dissociation, and the other showed how I felt after. The "before" was a stick figure with a big black whirlpool where the torso should be. The face was featureless. No eyes, ears, mouth, or nose. Just blankness. The limbs were drawn with perforated lines meant to represent the transient sensation I felt in them. There were no hands. No feet.

The "after" drawing looked more like a person. There was still an angry black void in my womb space, the part of my body it was hardest to connect with. But I had a torso. My limbs had materialized in full. My face had all of its features. My mouth was drawn into a serious straight line.

Standing in the grass, I wondered if dissociation was really such a bad thing. Even medical literature describes dissociation as an avoidance-based coping strategy. Dissociation has two benefits for prey animals: an animal that is disconnected from its body during an attack won't feel much pain, and a predator might leave its quarry alone if it thinks it's dead, allowing it to escape. But when I typed "why is it bad to dissociate?" into a search engine, the Internet informed me that too much dissociation can lead a person to passively go along with risky situations and prevent recovery. Apparently, one needs to feel their feelings to process them.

I sighed and wondered if humans haven't gone too far in their quest to define their personalities, if they've over-pathologized themselves in an attempt to explain away unusual or uncomfortable habits that nonetheless serve important functions.

It's a concern I share with thousands of clinicians. Before the fifth edition of the *DSM* was released, members of the American Psychiatric Association's Society for Humanistic Psychology published an open letter that highlighted several problems with the proposed psychiatric manual, including the lowering of diagnostic thresholds, which could lead to diagnostic hyperinflation and unnecessary treatment. Within a few days of the open letter's release, 1,500 mental health professionals had signed it. That number grew tenfold and included over fifty professional organizations. But their concerns went unaddressed.

Critics of the BPD diagnostic category have asserted that the label treats trauma responses as psychologically abnormal. In a 2023 *Journal of the Royal Society of Medicine* article, the authors argue that BPD is a "mushy blancmange diagnosis that simply embraces too much pathology to be of any real value." The authors wrote that true personality disorders are made up of characteristics and traits that generally don't change over time. BPD's "diagnostic criteria are not enduring personality traits but rather fluctuating symptoms and behaviours."

Maybe BPD isn't a personality disorder. Maybe it's just a set of reactions to unreliable early environments. Or a series of strategies people use to survive adverse experiences. Perhaps the symptoms we develop aren't an illness but a behavioural pattern that simply allows humans to persist in a range of conditions.

DANCING ON EGGSHELLS

The facilitators called them *fidgets*. Plastic Play-Doh containers in every shade of the rainbow, plum-coloured squishy stress balls, a kindergarten classroom's supply of markers and pencil crayons, and fuzzy pipe cleaners crowded a conference table so large it was jammed into the cramped room at a haphazard angle. The youngest person of the dozen or so gathered around the table was in their early twenties. Our emotional intelligence, however, was more reflective of the recommended age to play with the objects in front of us—three years old and above.

By 2018, I had sat in so many stuffy rooms across from so many doctors and counsellors their faces blended together in my memory. But, at twenty-eight, I had never tried group therapy, a form of treatment in which I was to discuss my feelings with a collection of my peers under a professional's supervision. I had assumed it was more efficient to address my problems with a clinician instead of someone who was also attempting to recover. How wrong I was.

In order to bypass the lengthy group therapy waiting list, it had been necessary for me to meet with a diagnostic psychiatrist—a hawkish woman who was meant to diagnose me in forty minutes. Her office was dark and windowless and compounded my exhaustion, which lingered after my brief stay in the emergency department. We had gone over my personal, medical, and family histories. In her notes about the session, the psychiatrist described my affect as "anxious, downcast, [and] reactive to content."

Ultimately, she agreed I would benefit from the three-month-long weekly group that was meant to help people with BPD develop dialectical behaviour therapy (DBT) skills—a fancy term for strategies that might slow the never-ending cycle of hospitalizations, self-harm, and agony people with the disorder experience.

"The skills group is also helpful for trauma," the psychiatrist said. "Which is how we should account for your symptoms."

"So, you don't think I have BPD?" I asked.

"You might," she said. She had capped her pen and winced. "But BPD is a tricky label. I think it's best we leave it out of your file for now."

I sank into the plush office chair. The clarity I had felt after Rick suggested a BPD diagnosis clouded.

"I'm going to refer your partner to the family program for loved ones of people with BPD," she continued.

I had managed to get referred to the support I needed, but this fear of labelling a person with a stigmatized diagnosis can act as a barrier to what resources are available to us (something I had to contend with when it came time to register my disability with the government).

Despite us sharing a diagnosis (official or otherwise), there were more incongruities than similarities among the members of the DBT skills group. Sure, we all had an aversion to the overhead fluorescents and insisted the lights be turned off so we could sit in the wintry afternoon gloom that crept through the windows. The people gathered around the table were largely under thirty years old. Half the group vanished at the break to blow heady smoke clouds into the traffic on College Street. Most of us were under- or unemployed, scraping by on freelance contracts, retail work, or Ontario Disability Support Program (ODSP) payments. But our differences were evident in our behaviours, which was surprising to me since our personalities were considered disordered in the same manner. Some of us were high-strung and moody. Others were passive and dependent. The minority practised sobriety. A few introverts hardly said a word so the extroverts overcame the silence by infusing the room with charm and humour. Some cried openly. Others stalked the hallways during the break in the two-hour sessions. I took to the therapeutic exercises contained within the hefty photocopied skills book and religiously filled out the urge-tracking diary cards with the vigour of a teacher's pet. Three people dropped out before the group's end.

BPD is a broad diagnosis that allows for countless variations of the disorder. The people in group therapy were as diverse in their presentations of BPD as the collection of colourful objects on the table we gathered around.

This diversity is why mental health professionals have long sought to refine the broad definition of BPD. There are said to be at least four subtypes of the disorder—petulant, discouraged, impulsive, and self-destructive. These subtypes were devised by Theodore Millon (though subsequent research has attempted to improve and refine these groups). According to one of the many BPD workbooks I invested in, learning about BPD subtypes can help an individual better understand their illness to move beyond it. But it was difficult to determine which subtype I belonged to because of my poor sense of self.

I recognized that aspects of my conduct aligned with impulsive BPD. People with this subtype are said to be charismatic, flirtatious, and engaging but struggle with risky and aggressive behaviours. People with petulant BPD are recognized by their severe mood swings, passive-aggressive attitudes, pessimism, and tendency to try to control others—a reflection of what I felt like on bad days. My history of self-harm, substance use, and suicide attempts situated me with the self-destructive subtype. But I also saw so much of myself in the discouraged, or quiet, BPD subtype. I was primarily driven by a fear of abandonment, had periods of being high-functioning or successful, and directed most of my emotions and aggression inward.

I tried to tease out the particulars of my disorder with group therapy members outside our sessions. It would prove as helpful as the treatment—if not more. It began when four of us shuffled to the Tim Hortons at College and Spadina when we weren't quite ready to wrap up our conversation but our cigarette fingers stung from the glacial wind. It became a regular habit.

We'd grab a table by an electric fireplace that spat counterfeit flames if we were lucky. Usually, we ended up by the bathrooms. It was always hectic in that particular Tim Hortons. It teemed with students from the University of Toronto, people from CAMH's emergency department, and teens who had spent the day shopping in Kensington Market's overpriced vintage shops. In that chaos, we felt like we belonged. We swapped our life stories with the thrill of new lovers who realize they share the same star sign, buoyed by each other's energy and interest. We set our trauma side by side to see if we could find the throughline that connected our motley experiences to our medical diagnosis. We tried to figure out who we were.

George, Jay, Odessa, and I called ourselves (and our subsequent group chat) the Breakfast Club, after the 1985 John Hughes film in which a disparate group of teenagers bond when they're forced into close quarters for a day-long detention.

We extended additional invitations to two more group members, Steph and a woman I'll call Margaret, over the next few sessions. At first glance, it didn't seem we had much in common. We were all in different places in our lives, came from different backgrounds, and had different interests, but the glue that cemented our friendship was dynamic discussions of our lives with BPD. We compared self-harm and substance-use histories, which antidepressants and anti-anxiety medications helped reduce our symptoms, whether our turbulent adolescent years and broken childhoods were a symptom or the source of our personality disorder. We lingered in the coffee shop until the sky stripped itself of its light.

Winter thawed into spring. We completed group treatment. Life was slowly returning to the city, but the group members were still dormant. We had learned healthier coping strategies through DBT, but many of our symptoms persisted. We still needed support. We turned to each other. Our conversations moved beyond coffee shops to Margaret's crystal-filled apartment in the west end, to Jay's apartment in the Village before they moved back to their hometown, and to the Cabbagetown apartment that George and Steph eventually shared. That summer, we met in Trinity Bellwoods, a park bustling with hipsters drinking local beers, dogs chasing frisbees, and errant footballs colliding with unsuspecting picnickers.

"Did I tell you guys I was looking for symbols for my artwork and I figured out what animal would best represent BPD?" Steph asked. She took a drag of her cigarette and winced against the smoke. Her unlined and freckled face didn't betray her tumultuous history, which included moving to Toronto from Halifax just to find treatment.

We shook our heads.

"The hog-nosed snake," Steph said. "They're very small but when they're threatened, they pretend to be a cobra. They'll hiss at you and bump you with their nose, but they won't actually bite. When they realize they can't scare you, they roll over, belly up, stick their tongue out, and pretend to die. They stay immobilized, but every so often they peek out of one eye to see if they're safe."

"That's pretty good," Jay said.

Odessa passed around a Tupperware container filled with her homemade lemon squares. Odessa's Barbadian grandmother had treated her childhood tempers with baking like mine had. Our grandmothers were on to something. Baking was one of the recommended self-soothing activities we learned in therapy.

"How's living with your parents going?" George asked Jay, who had moved back to their hometown.

"Any plans to move back to the city?" I asked.

Jay's lips, painted an icy blue, stretched into a grimace. "Not right now. Part of me wants to, but I don't feel strong enough to live on my own."

"I get that," Odessa said. "I don't feel strong enough to be working right now."

"Are you still at the sex shop?" I asked.

Odessa nodded and swallowed more lemon square. "The customers are all right, but the manager is a smug nightmare. I want to quit so bad."

"You could try ODSP, but it's stressful. After I pay my bills, I have hardly anything to live on," Steph said.

We spotted Margaret's slim figure crossing the park. "Sorry I'm late, guys," she said once she closed the distance between us. "My tattoo appointment took longer than I expected." Margaret was covered in tattoos inspired by pop culture—a strategy she recommended to minimize self-harm.

George took Margaret into his muscly arms. "How are you doing, babe?"

She sighed and shrugged. "I'm going to really focus on working on me now that my ex and I aren't doing the confusing 'friends' thing."

"So proud of you, girl," George said. "I was the same way until I met you guys in the DBT skills group."

I couldn't parse the subtypes of my friends with BPD. Like *The Breakfast Club*'s archetypes—the athlete, the nerd, the criminal, the princess, and the basket case—BPD subtypes aren't clean or without overlap. Each one of us was the discouraged borderline, the impulsive borderline, the petulant borderline, and the self-destructive borderline.

✳

On February 8, 2021, George sent a meme to the group chat of a skeleton wearing fairy wings and a tutu that read "When you're dead inside, but your best friend needs emotional support."

Each day bled into the next during Toronto's seemingly unending COVID-19 lockdowns. Our WhatsApp group chat was my most consistent source of levity and empathy amid the unrelenting monotony of household chores, writing deadlines, and screaming cats. Its profile image featured a distressed Aaron Paul as Jesse Pinkman from *Breaking Bad* overlaid with the words *intensity intensifies*. The most succinct description of BPD.

"Today's personal mood board is brought to you by being called out by your search history," Odessa wrote a few weeks later. The screencap she shared included the queries "Can you overdose on Zoloft?," "How to get your life together," "COVID-19 Toronto," and "carrot muffins whole wheat."

People with BPD are known for their unstable relationships, which can affect our ability to sustain long-term connections. Yet years after the DBT skills group ended, George, Jay, Odessa, and I nurtured and maintained our impromptu support space. Steph had taken a break due to political disagreements, and Margaret had found a different support group better suited to her needs—sad losses but moves we understood as necessary for their recoveries. The remaining members with the disorder shared another important connection: we all fell under the 2SLGTBQIA+ umbrella.

BPD is thought to be more common among the 2SLGTBQIA+ community than among heterosexual people. A 2008 study found people with BPD were 75 per cent more likely to identify as gay or bisexual than comparison subjects with other personality disorders.

However, 9 per cent of people surveyed reported having intimate relationships with the same sex without identifying as gay or bisexual. The authors noted that people with BPD might be reluctant to label themselves 2SLGTBQIA+ due to social stigma. The Breakfast Club had been making good strides in our recovery journeys. Then the pandemic hit. New anxieties blossomed, panic attacks returned, and despair wrapped its familiar tendrils around us. We weren't alone. Sixty-one per cent of people with pre-existing mental illness reported deteriorating mental health during the first six months of the pandemic. Luckily, we could turn to each other for support. We shared a penchant for coping with trauma through gallows humour. Despite our differences, we seemed to inherently know how to comfort each other—a deeply felt linguistic shorthand that developed effortlessly.

The pandemic provoked distinct reactions in each of us. Jay struggled with anxiety, paranoia around getting sick, and fears about the future. "Trying to calm the screaming lizard brain," they admitted in March 2020. I reminded Jay that they were young and likely to recover if they got sick. (Those were more optimistic days.) Never one to miss a beat, George jumped in with a cheeky "Or win the lottery and finally return to the void."

Odessa was grappling with an anxiety disorder brought on by the pandemic: agoraphobia—the fear of crowds, public spaces, or being trapped in places it's hard to escape from. "I'm going through that cycle of 'let's get motivated, work out maybe, and figure out what I want to do with my life that doesn't make me want to die,' and 'I'd rather flay off my skin than become a functioning human.'"

"We're in a pandemic," I said. "Fuck functioning. I had a panic attack in a parking lot this week." Odessa may have felt aimless, but she dedicated a significant amount of her energy to advocating for 2SLGTBQIA+ and BIPOC communities.

The accessibility of the group chat was its greatest feature even prior to COVID-19. Corralling people with BPD for an in-person hang is a bit like wrangling cats. Our availability is dependent on our moods, which are as unpredictable as the weather. The group chat became a virtual communal meeting ground we could access on our own terms. After the city's public queer spaces were deemed non-essential and closed, it was one of the few safe places we could visit.

And it was important for us to band together. 2SLGTBQIA+ people are more likely to face prejudice, social rejection, discrimination, and isolation. Such stigma is an extreme form of invalidation. Invalidation, or the rejection of a person's experiences, emotions, beliefs, and actions, is thought to be a factor that causes BPD. There's evidence that clinicians participate in this stigma and may be predisposed to provide a BPD diagnosis to people who come from sexual minorities. For example, men who have difficulty coming out are more likely to be diagnosed with the disorder. This suggests that clinicians might be more likely to pair stigmatized illnesses with stigmatized sexual identities, assigning labels to populations they don't fully understand.

Perhaps that's why we turned to each other for help more often than turning to traditional mental health care. Jay best captured why the group chat was such an important safe haven for us, using the Greek myth of Atlas, condemned to hold up Earth for eternity:

"It was that he had to do it alone, which is the true punishment. We have to carry a lot around. It's only really punishing once we are left to handle it all alone."

✳

"You have to show the world we're not monsters," George said. "We're just reacting to stress the only way we know how to."

Pandemic restrictions had eased. In the aftermath of the breakup that led him to the hospital and eventually the Breakfast Club, George had met his new partner, Neill. We were hanging out in the cozy Cabbagetown apartment they shared. I was visiting to deliver the news that I was planning to write a book about BPD.

"My biggest issue is the complete misrepresentation of what BPD is," he continued. "I've read books about the disorder that describe it as this awful horrible thing that just wreaks havoc on people with BPD and their loved ones."

"*Walking on Eggshells*?" I asked.

"Yes! What an awful book. I couldn't make it to the end. It was so depressing."

It was a variation of a conversation we'd had before. George was pursuing a Ph.D. in psychology, specializing in BPD, in hopes he could help treat and prevent the disorder in others. Our shared professional interest led to thorough discussions about medical stigma, attachment styles, and mistrust as it related to BPD, which grew into one of the roots that grounded our enduring friendship.

"I don't want to romanticize the disorder, but I want to focus on some of its positives or strengths," I said. I took a swig from my beer and inched closer to the roasting fireplace that interrupted our conversation with hisses and pops.

"Totally! The intense happiness, how quick we are to pick up on emotional cues"—George stopped to arch an eyebrow—"how amazing we are in bed."

"I don't think that's been proven empirically yet." The beer bubbles had gone to my brain, and I lapsed into a spasm of giggles.

George and I dealt with our fair share of mental health setbacks during the pandemic, but navigating our romantic relationships during lockdown proved the most challenging. I was six years into my relationship and George had been with his partner for more than a year, but the maladaptive behaviours our upbringings ingrained into us made it agonizing to communicate our feelings and emotions to our loved ones. Simple disagreements ballooned into hours of panic, upset, dissociation, and impulsive behaviours like self-harm. We had no road map to navigate interpersonal friction because we hadn't been exposed to healthy relationships. Growing up, we had to fundamentally alter our behaviours to survive unsafe environments. Luckily, we could turn to each other to brainstorm strategies to improve our relationship dynamics.

I had never been very good at friendship. At least, not the enduring friendships other people had. I moved around so much that my elementary school days were a haze of young faces. I regularly confused the little girls at my desk clumps whose hair was carefully brushed and braided by their stay-at-home mothers while mine hung loose and tangled. In grade two, I went to four different schools before Christmas. I ingratiated myself into social groups easily enough. I rarely ate lunch alone, and if I had to, I instead avoided it altogether by stalking the streets that surrounded whichever school I found myself at. But my friendships trailed off like unfinished sentences as soon as the moving truck pulled out of our driveway. The cracks in my social skills would eventually trip up my companions if my family stuck around a place for more than a year or two. I'd commit some tactless blunder that alienated me, like clinging too hard and spending every weekend with one friend until they inevitably got sick of me. Or my impulsive mouth got me in trouble. It didn't matter though. There were always new friends to be made down the road.

The fear of being an imposition overpowered my urge to connect as I aged and became more aware of my personality's quirks. I learned Morse code so I could tap SOS on my friends' flesh and ask for help without taking up any verbal space. If the friend didn't pick up on my distress signal (none of them ever did), our relationship proceeded undamaged by my insatiable need for assistance. In high school, my friendships were tainted by transactions. Constant couch-surfing meant I was a steady drain on resources even when I tried to stay small.

My experience aligns with a 2021 scoping review of friendships among adolescents with BPD. The authors found that interpersonal relationships were typically disrupted, had unclear or permeable boundaries, and tended to be overdependent. Jealousy toward friends was common—teenagers with BPD were more likely to demand exclusivity in their friendships, which was proposed as an early indicator of the disorder in addition to a heightened sensitivity to rejection. These peer relationships in people with BPD, the authors noted, could be building upon troubled parent-child relationships.

By adulthood, I had learned how to better navigate social cues. I made a few lasting friends at university and at work, but I always felt like the new kid—that spending time with me was an act of charity. I was obliged to mirror new friends' interests, wits, or hobbies because as far as I was concerned, I was just lucky to have people who wanted to be around me. I was certain that history would repeat itself. That my friendships would fade in the rear-view mirror.

These patterns didn't emerge in my friendships with people with BPD. My friendships with people who shared my way of moving through the world were free of the social anxiety and pretense that pervaded so many of my relationships.

"From a personal perspective, BPD has probably been one of the best things in my life in a lot of aspects," George said after he returned from fetching two more beers from the fridge. "It is a consistent and constant challenge, an opportunity to learn, to think in a completely different way, to better myself, to understand how others think, to be more patient with them, to pick up on social cues a lot easier, and be there for people."

My face melted into an easy smile. George was right. BPD had taught me to be aware of my emotions and relationship patterns in ways most people weren't. But he had also grasped the heart of my book's intentions as clearly as if he held them in his hand.

The summer I signed my book contract, George brought me a souvenir from his Serbian family's holiday as a thank-you for watching Neill's cat. It was a small woodblock painting of the Croatian coastline. A cherry-red sun sat in the corner of an azure sky and shone down on a lighthouse that towered over colourful buildings.

On the sand were words painted in a black script: "If your ship doesn't come in, swim out to it."

I found my ships in other people with BPD. And I was happy to swim out to them.

✳

Tracey and I sat on a bench in St. James Park in Toronto surrounded by newly unfurled leaves. Her eighty-pound service dog was smushed between us. Hot dog breath mingled with notes of tulips and snowdrops in the soft breeze. A bearded guy walked by and asked us if we could spare fifty dollars, but I only had a toonie. We joked about post-pandemic inflation.

"So, did your BPD come from, like, capital-T traumas?" Tracey asked once the man drifted off.

I paused and petted the dog's velvety golden head. "I guess it's all relative, but I think so. There are a few incidents that I can point out—the same ones that return to haunt me every so often—that definitely had an impact."

"That's interesting. I don't feel like mine did. I mean, there was a bunch of small-t stuff but nothing concrete I can point to."

"Well, Linehan was the same way," I said. "It's the whole tulip-raised-in-a-rose-garden concept. The invalidation can be enough."

I didn't have to explain to Tracey that one of the proposed causes of BPD is early invalidation, or that Linehan described the concept in her memoir, *Building a Life Worth Living*, with a gardening metaphor. Tracey already knew that Linehan wrote, "Mother saw me as a tulip and desperately wanted to make me into a rose.

She thought I'd be happier as a rose. But I did not have what it took to be a rose, not then and not now." It's an analogy Linehan would later use to advise her clients with BPD, "If you're a tulip, don't try to be a rose. You have to find a tulip garden."

Tracey and I met the way everyone did during the pandemic—online. We were accepted into a fellowship at Yale University's program for recovery and community health, which fostered leadership skills in people with lived experience of mental illness. Our introductory session on Webex (a more secure Zoom-like platform) included an opportunity to introduce ourselves to the faculty and co-fellows. I heard from people who wanted to create mobile mental health units for young people of colour, mail-based art projects to engage marginalized people living with mental illness during the pandemic, and a magazine dedicated to publishing people who identified as mad or neurodivergent. I had hoped someone would mention BPD during the introductions. By the time my turn came, no one had. I cleared my throat, plastered on my bravest smile, and announced that I both lived with and wrote about the disorder. The chat box on the right-hand side of the screen filled up with others who were diagnosed. One or two people who had gone before me turned their mics back on to say they also had BPD but were too nervous to disclose it due to the stigma associated with the label. Tracey was among them.

"Do you mind if I ask if you're in treatment right now?" Tracey said. Her pup froze and snapped his head to the left to glare at a squirrel scaling a nearby tree.

I told her I was still seeing the therapist I'd been assigned when I began the skills group while she distracted her dog from chewing its leash. But I was lucky—publicly funded mental health support is rarely long-term. The odds a person will connect with their counsellor in a way that's conducive to meaningful healing feel only slightly better than winning the lottery.

"I was thinking I could use some extra support right now," Tracey said. "But I'm so burnt out on traditional mental health care."

I understood her wariness. Around the time Tracey and I met in the park, the government of Canada announced changes to its medical assistance in dying (MAID) law. The amended law would grant people with depression, bipolar disorder, schizophrenia, PTSD, or personality disorders like BPD the right to die with medical aid.

Framed as a form of compassionate care, there were already signs that the law might replace efforts to create equitable access to mental health support and develop meaningful treatment strategies for poorly understood mental health conditions, and that it would instead entrench the idea that certain mental illnesses were untreatable. It was simply a lot cheaper to assist a person with mental illness in dying than it was to heal them.

In 2021, three United Nations human rights experts flagged that the amendment appeared to violate the UN's Universal Declaration of Human Rights and could "have a potentially discriminatory impact on persons with disabilities." There were unconfirmed whispers that mental health helplines in the country had begun to recommend MAID to callers who were in distress. Unlike other countries that offer euthanasia, Canadian doctors are free to inform their patients that death is one of their health care options, and patients aren't required to exhaust other treatments before applying to die.

The fear of human rights violations was warranted. In April 2022, a fifty-one-year-old Ontario woman became the first person to be granted MAID for multiple chemical sensitivities, a chronic environmental illness, after her search for affordable housing free from cigarette smoke failed. "The government sees me as expendable trash, a complainer, useless, and a pain in the ass," the woman said in a video filmed before her death that was shared with CTV. In December 2022, Canada's justice minister David Lametti announced that more time might be necessary to ensure the country's assisted dying measures were prudent. Exercising the right to die is a personal decision, but death shouldn't be the only option available to people who have fallen through the gaps in a social safety net stretched to its seams.

The dog was ready for a ramble. Tracey and I followed him through the grass to the copper-roofed cathedral that cast shadows over the park.

It took me a long time to find a garden with the growing conditions I thrived in. I knew that there was a risk I'd lose some of my favourite flowers once my tulip garden grew big enough—up to 10 per cent of people with BPD die by suicide, a fiftyfold increase compared to the general population. I hadn't anticipated that the government would carry out the culling.

✳

I had always dreamed of an entirely virtual event when I worked as an event producer. An event where I didn't have to deal with the crippling anxiety that held hands with overstimulation as I tried to navigate confusing social cues and worked in overdrive to limit my impulsive urges at boozy receptions choked with lecherous egos willing to take advantage of the sick and the naive.

Virtual events were a reality during the pandemic. In 2022, I was invited to participate in a panel about life with BPD. My rotund cat softly snored beneath the window beside me. My bookshelves filled with the voices of writers who had made me feel less alone over the years watched over my shoulder. Without the pressures of an in-person production, there was no quiet sobbing in a venue bathroom while panels were underway.

The event began. The producer had limited the audience to an intimate size. I suspected she did so for more than just the panelists' comfort. I think she was trying to create a space free from the poison Amber Heard's alleged BPD diagnosis generated during the Johnny Depp defamation lawsuit, which at that time was underway.

While the producer delivered her opening remarks, it hit me that I had spent most of the previous year in digital spaces almost exclusively occupied by people who lived with BPD or serious mental illness. I had never felt more comfortable. So much more patience and empathy were practised by the people in those places: the extra few minutes to finish up an important thought even if a meeting had gone over time, permission to keep the camera off when facing the world and those in it was too much, the ability to be honest when a panic attack interrupted the day's forward march. It was a way of life that may strike a certain type of person as weakness, but there was strength in our vulnerability. In a way, people with BPD *were* like eggshells. Possible to crack when smacked against the lip of a ceramic bowl but capable of withstanding great weights when the burden was evenly distributed.

I showed up in spaces where those with the disorder and mental illness congregated. I plucked my people out like fabric scraps, which I braided together to form a complete support system. But I was only able to find my community because I was open about my diagnosis. That isn't the case for many people with BPD. But perhaps if BPD were framed in less stigmatizing terms more people would publicly identify with the disorder. In a gentler world, spaces occupied by people with BPD would be bountiful and easy to access. People with the disorder would be able to look to others who have BPD and sidestep the stigma so prevalent in the mental health sector and the general public. We could strategize with others who had first-hand knowledge of BPD instead of those who had merely studied it. Since the disorder hinges so much on emotion, it's vital that the people who discuss it on a public stage know what it feels like. As one person who attended the event noted, the particulars of life with the disorder hit differently when a person gets to "listen and learn *with* people with BPD and not learn *about* them."

What that attendee recognized was one of the guiding principles of peer support. Peer support is an oft-overlooked form of mentorship and emotional aid delivered to people with mental illness by people with their own lived experience. I learned through the Yale fellowship that the practice involves a lot of active listening to others who are struggling with their mental health, offering advice or empathy informed by the peer supporter's experiences, and encouraging people to use their unique strengths to support their recovery. Peer supporters didn't treat mental illness but modelled how to live with mental health challenges effectively. When people saw others who lived with mental illness thrive, it gave them hope that they could recover and live a meaningful life too.

Peer support can be informal, like the help the Breakfast Club provides to one another or the work George and I did to support others who lived with the disorder. But it can also be a semi-formal role within the health care system that involves aid delivered by a trained and paid peer supporter. Peer work can happen in conjunction with or separately from clinical treatment, and it may be one-on-one or in group settings. It's primarily available through mental health organizations, but peers in support roles can also be found in institutions, such as hospitals or universities. Required experience or accreditation varies widely.

Within the Western mental health system, peer support dates back to the late eighteenth century, when Bicêtre Hospital in Paris hired former patients as hospital staff. In a 1793 letter, Jean-Baptiste Pussin, the facility's governor and a former patient, wrote that recovered patients were "better suited to this demanding work because they are usually more gentle, honest, and humane."

In Canada, models of peer support have been available since at least the early 1940s, when Alcoholics Anonymous started crossing the border from the U.S. In 1971, the Mental Patients Association of Vancouver, the country's first peer-run support organization, was founded in British Columbia following Canada's deinstitutionalization movement, which advocated for community-based care for people with mental illness. By the 1980s, former patients in Toronto launched several community initiatives like drop-in centres, second-hand stores, and the magazine *Phoenix Rising*. The role of peer supporters became more formalized within health policy but was met with mixed responses and often fell at the mercy of budget cuts during this period.

Some studies show that peer support services are equally as effective as similar services provided by non-peer professionals and have a more positive impact on levels of hope, empowerment, and quality of life. The Mental Health Commission of Canada found the benefits of peer support also included reduced hospitalization rates, less isolation and symptom distress, and lower costs for the health care sector.

This last point is significant. The economic burden of mental illness in Canada is estimated to be 51 billion dollars per year. In a 2005 study conducted in Ontario, people who received peer support were discharged from the hospital an average of 116 days sooner than those who didn't, which resulted in considerable savings. A 2018 *Psychiatric Times* article illustrated that peer support is a "win-win situation for resource-strapped systems." People living with mental illness receive support that instills hope and assists in their recovery journey, people with lived experience of mental illness are employed in roles that support their well-being, and the mental health system gains an effective and trained workforce.

For people with BPD, peer supporters with the diagnosis can validate our experiences. In a 2020 qualitative study about peer work, one of the people interviewed noted, "I, personally, would prefer someone (a consumer peer worker) with BPD. Not another diagnosis . . . a lot of my own experience with BPD could only really be understood by somebody else with BPD."

When it was time for the panel to end, I didn't feel relieved like I used to when an in-person event finished, ready to order the largest bowl of off-menu spaghetti possible from a hotel bar before I kicked off my flats and collapsed into a plush armchair, the tension in my mind at last loose and formless like an elastic band that had been stretched too far. Instead, I was able to easily navigate an experience I used to find overwhelming because I had been surrounded by my peers. The panel's audience talked about how validated they felt, which helps support emotional regulation—one of the central difficulties for people with the disorder. Family members who attended were going to exercise more empathy and patience toward their loved ones with BPD now that they were empowered with more information. I was able to give others hope, which reinforced my own strength.

For a long time, I didn't imagine anything positive could come out of my personality disorder. In solitude, it seemed I was cursed to cycle continuously between silos in the mental health sector. It was excruciatingly lonely. I didn't feel so fragile once I was among people who had walked a similar path. My friendships with others with BPD taught me that it is okay to take up space in the lives of people I care about. That it is enough to be myself.

EXQUISITELY SENSITIVE

Darkness snuggled up against the windows of Neill's Cabbagetown apartment. A crackling fire cast the living room in a warm glow. Aegean lounge music played through the television speakers. We had recently marked the one-year anniversary of COVID-19's extended stay-at-home orders.

My partner, M., and I had traversed the wintry city masked in KN95s for a double date with our bubble, George and his partner, Neill. When we came in, George hugged me in a way customary to people with BPD—like they've reached into your body to cradle your soul.

But my goal for the occasion was loftier than mere socialization. I had been interviewing people with BPD from group therapy about their relationships for a newsletter I write about life with the disorder. It was time to talk to our non-borderline partners. Specifically, to M. and Neill.

George, M., and I settled onto an expansive grey couch while Neill doled out cans of beer.

"The conversation shouldn't be too daunting," I said. "I'd like to discuss how our relationships are unique—our sensitivity and intensity, perhaps—and some of the strategies you use to navigate our partnerships."

What I didn't tell the group was that I had a secret tertiary reason for the conversation beyond my literary ambitions or earnest hopes that publishing parts of the discussion might result in less stigma for people who lived with BPD. I was in a bad place. The pandemic had compounded my more gruelling symptoms—panic attacks, self-harm, and sweeping mood swings. My self-worth was suffering. I could no longer fathom what strengths (if any) I brought to the table. I smiled at the people who loved me enough to let me excavate their insights with a swelling hope that they could remind me of my redeeming qualities.

George, always wordlessly in tune with my apprehensions, squeezed my kneecap. "Don't worry," he said while the firelight danced across his face. "It's going to be great."

As I'm writing this book in 2023, reducing stigma around mental illness is all the rage—particularly for the "softer" diagnoses like depression and anxiety that intensified for many people due to the pandemic. Governments, universities, media organizations, telecommunications giants, and even individuals are discussing mental health more than ever. Yet BPD, like many of the "scarier" mental health diagnoses, remains a highly condemned disorder thought to come with few compensatory attributes. However, despite people with BPD's impaired functioning, medical professionals have long noticed that people with the disorder possess innate gifts like increased empathy, high intelligence, artistic talent, and strong self-awareness.

American psychologist and psychoanalyst Alan Krohn was the first to make note of these gifts in a 1974 paper. He detailed a phenomenon he called *borderline empathy*, an ability to accurately read the emotional states of others. His paper described a young woman with BPD who struggled with drug use, exhibited strange behaviour, and was unable to cope when separated from her mother. But once she was hospitalized, she demonstrated a keen insight into those around her. She had "a remarkable sensitivity to turmoil in other patients and staff." She described a strange energy coming from a staff member who, it later turned out, was in distress. The young woman explained that it looked like the staff member was seeing someone get killed. "He was in fact preoccupied with thoughts of brutalities he witnessed in battle."

Another person with BPD consistently put into words their therapists' private thoughts and feelings just as the therapist was having them. Krohn noted that people with the disorder were likely to provoke "deep confronting interpretation[s]" of a therapist's personal inner conflicts. People with BPD were able to pick up on the feelings of clinicians who were trained to minimize their emotional expressions. Krohn had tapped into a paradox. The empathic paradox, or borderline empathy paradox, is defined as enhanced empathy in spite of impaired interpersonal function. Some people with BPD could recognize and mirror the most subtle emotional states of the people around them, but this ability failed to smooth the path for the development of lasting personal relationships.

Three years later, psychiatrists from the Topeka Veterans Administration Hospital published a paper that attempted to explain people with BPD's sensitivity to the inner worlds of others, particularly those with whom they had "symbiotic-like" relationships. Authors Linnea Carter and Donald Rinsley drew upon Krohn's work and research by psychiatrist Edward R. Shapiro to hypothesize that heightened empathy first occurred during early childhood development—specifically between the stage when an infant is completely dependent on their mother and a reciprocal sensitivity to non-verbal cues and the stage when a child begins to develop a sense of themself and an understanding of their mother as an individual. When a child fixated between these stages, tuning into their caregiver's inner world allowed them to keep a consistent view of inconsistent mothers. Such children developed an overly intense awareness of their environment. In adults and teenagers with BPD, this awareness presented as a "unique ability to empathize with others." At the time, the authors believed the empathy paradox represented a prolonged manifestation of the efforts people with BPD had engaged in as small children.

Derision bled into early research about enhanced empathy in people with BPD. Our perceptiveness was often framed as a deficit in disguise. Or a power used to infuriate the people who treated us. In a 1978 literature review of people with the disorder, Shapiro wrote of our peculiar empathetic abilities: "When frustrated or projecting their anger in therapy . . . borderline patients may utilize this intuition to provoke a response . . . to justify their distrust and may then destroy, devalue, or reject all the therapist has to offer." Shapiro acknowledged the precision with which people with BPD could pick up on others' unconscious impulses but described the group as having little ability to recognize healthy relationships with reality or when another person was repressing their true feelings by behaving opposite to how they felt.

For a few years, interest in borderline empathy research seemingly waned. It was replaced by analyses of the families of people with BPD, treatment manuals, and discussions of the various psychic failings people with the disorder experienced. In 1986, the thread was picked up again. Researchers from McGill University conducted a study to provide empirical evidence of borderline empathy. Authors Hallie Frank and Norman Hoffman determined women with BPD were "significantly more sensitive" to positive and negative non-verbal communication than the control groups. The authors analyzed research about families of people with BPD and found that neglect from both caregivers was more strongly linked to borderline empathetic abilities than inconsistent or symbiotic mothering. The authors conceded that people with BPD may add projections onto their empathic insights, but "their basic perceptions are often accurate."

Two years later, a study in the *British Journal of Medical Psychology* determined that people with BPD had stronger empathetic abilities than people with schizophrenia or neuroses. What's more, they were as insightful as the therapists involved in the study, who likely had more knowledge of the people they were treating than the people with BPD did.

Around this time, researchers tried to establish the qualities of people with BPD who were likely to fare well over the course of their lifetime. During a presentation at the American Psychiatric Association's 150th annual meeting, psychiatrist Michael H. Stone introduced a list of characteristics that influenced if a person with the disorder was likely to improve with time. Stone found that people with BPD who had better recovery outcomes were more likely to be highly intelligent (with an IQ higher than 130), possess unusual artistic talent, and have "obsessive-compulsive" characteristics that strengthened self-discipline and the ability to maintain a work-life balance. Disturbingly, women with BPD who were physically attractive also had better recovery odds.

Mental health professionals have noted additional strengths in people with the disorder. Researchers from Germany devised a simple test to measure self-awareness. Female participants were given the choice between a seat that faced a mirror and one that didn't. The participants were asked to indicate if their choice was intentional after they made it. As the researchers predicted, people with BPD often chose a chair that didn't face the mirror; however, it was their intentions that differed strongly from the rest of the participants. Ninety per cent of people with BPD noted their chair choice was intentional, whereas only 27 per cent of healthy controls made a conscious decision. People with BPD might be more conscious of intent than the average person.

In their 2007 book, *The Borderline Personality Disorder Survival Guide*, authors Alexander Chapman and Kim Gratz describe people with BPD as "dramatic, exciting, and charismatic." They submitted that this is why television and film industries were interested in portraying characters with the disorder, yet they rarely depicted the nuances of BPD, which contributed to public stigma. This could also be why so few people choose to identify publicly with the disorder— to live their reality out loud. Yet those who do have undeniable gifts:

actor and comedian Pete Davidson, singer Madison Beer, writer Susanna Kaysen, model and actress Madison Bailey, former professional football player Brandon Marshall, author and playwright Kate Bornstein, actor and comedian Darrell Hammond, and singer Sinead O'Connor.

Perhaps this list would be even longer if mental health experts explored the gifts that came with the disorder in more depth. Or at least made an effort to include mention of these gifts in places where people with BPD seek out information about the disorder. Unfortunately, people with BPD are unlikely to learn anything positive about our diagnosis without an incredibly deep dive into the literature. We might see pitying looks, hear the sharp sound of breath sucked through teeth, or read a laundry list of catastrophic symptoms like I did when I was being diagnosed. With time, it's easy to internalize the disorder's negative prognosis, the dire research reports, and the nasty quips on social media. Hopelessness pervades. Harmful symptoms surface. A person with BPD is bound to wander into a dark night of the soul when no glimmer of hope shines on the horizon.

After dinner, George, Neill, M., and I pushed back from the candlelit table, patting our bellies and sighing. I can't be specific about what we ate—so many of my memories from the pandemic blur together. The room smelled of fire smoke. The lights were dim and the cat circled our chair legs on the hunt for food scraps or pets. Outside, tiny snowflakes rushed to the ground in swarms.

"How's everyone feeling?" I asked once our drinks were refreshed. "Ready to get into it?"

Neill smiled shyly and leaned to the side of his chair to pet his cat. "Now is as good a time as any."

I retrieved the printout of questions I'd devised ahead of time, smoothed out the creases in the paper, and placed it and my phone, set to record, between wine glasses and food crumbs. I cleared my throat. My eyes zeroed in on a pleasant question. "What are some of the best aspects of having a partner with BPD?" I asked.

Neill folded his hands on the table. His brow creased. He angled himself toward George. "You're sometimes more in tune with a reaction, an emotion, or an energy before it's happened."

George's eyes sparkled. He interlaced his fingers into Neill's. "Thanks, handsome."

"Like the other day," Neill continued, "we were at your place and you kept asking if I was okay. I wasn't. I just didn't know it yet. As soon as I left your place, I was in tears. Something was building all day, but you caught onto it and knew it was there before I did." Neill looked up at M. and me and smirked. "It's a nice little warning system."

"I just wanted to fix what was bothering you," George said.

"What about you?" I asked M.

M. nodded his head from side to side, the way he often did when he was carefully considering his answer. "I think people with BPD are a little more in touch with what it means to be alive, what it is that is necessary from life, and are focused on getting it, which is a bit atypical for the human experience. There are a lot of people who are just resigned to shades of grey. Sometimes, people with BPD only want to paint in colour. To be that person's partner—you just stand back and revel."

"Yes!" Neill said. "And it's noticeable when that colour is dull or when there's a cloud over it. It changes its luminosity. A grey day can get into their heads—the colour is there but only at one or two per cent. It's noticeable when that colour is full throttle. It's a changing energy, a changing liveliness in their expression, eyes, their description of a memory."

"It's interesting you bring that up because George and I talk a lot about the importance of colour in our lives," I said.

"We don't see colour as brightly when we're sad," George explained. "But the whole world shines when everything is fine."

I nodded. The hues in the living room had warmed. The candle's flame, a pale yellow when the dinner began, blazed orange as it licked away at melting wax. The dull red in M.'s plaid shirt had brightened into a vibrant cherry.

The link between our emotions and colours was likely just a case of synesthesia, the blending of senses, which is a common phenomenon experienced by neurodivergent people or people with mental illness. But our empathic talents might be unique to people with BPD. In chapter six of *Psychological Mindedness: A Contemporary Understanding*, authors Lee Crandall Park and Thomas J. Park noted that people who develop BPD "frequently have a special talent or gift." Based on research they conducted in 1992, the authors determined that people with BPD were gifted when it came to personal intelligence or the ability to notice the moods, temperaments, motivations, and intentions of others.

The 1992 clinical study was conducted on outpatient men and women with BPD. Seventy-four per cent of people with BPD met the study's definition of giftedness. Every participant with BPD in the study was considered as having an intense preoccupation with and/or talented access to others' feelings. This suggested to the authors that high levels of personal intelligence in people with BPD were abundant. The study determined that histories of neglect and chronic verbal or psychological abuse were common in gifted people with BPD. But a history of trauma wasn't enough to explain these strengths. People with other personality disorders also experienced a lot of neglect and verbal abuse, but fewer were considered gifted—just 13 per cent.

The authors found additional references in literature to people with BPD's ability to involve and influence others, including their tendency to "evoke seriously disruptive staff conflicts in which one or more [hospital] staff members passionately protect the [person with BPD] as a 'helpless waif' requiring nurturance."

And nowhere were these gifts more apparent or powerful than in the therapist's office. People with BPD were described as "exquisitely sensitive to the daily emotional state of the therapist, his tone of voice, and nonverbal messages conveyed by gestures and body posture." From Otto Kernberg's *Psychodynamic Psychotherapy of Borderline Patients*, a rather concerning look at psychiatric practice: "Uncannily, borderline patients seem to sense the therapist's vulnerability and may choose the exact moment when the therapist wishes the patient dead to announce a suicide plan." People with BPD were represented as "remarkably appealing" and even seductive.

In Park and Park's 1992 study, they described a person with BPD who sensed her therapist's feelings of unexpressed pessimism toward her prospects. She turned this perception around on the therapist to make him feel as hopeless as possible. Another person with the disorder corrected her therapist's treatment approach without warning. "It doesn't help me if you feel sorry for me," she said. "It throws me off and I can't help trying to make you feel that way even more. It's like an addiction, to make you have a feeling for me." The authors wrote that an exceptional degree of personal intelligence must be involved to allow a person with BPD to pick up on the feelings of their therapist and intensify them while both remained unaware of the persuasive dynamics.

Under optimal circumstances, the authors argued, infants with these gifts would grow up to become distinctly successful in their relationships and careers instead of developing BPD. Similar habits had been observed in rhesus monkeys. When rhesus monkeys were bred to be anxious or fearful in new conditions and highly aware of their environment, they maintained this tendency into adulthood. When the anxious monkeys were raised by nurturing foster mothers, they became the most skilled and dominant members of their peer groups.

Children have to maintain the sense that their caregivers are capable and safe. In circumstances where abuse was threatening enough to interfere with children's healthy development, infants' intuitive talents were directed entirely to understanding and resolving feelings about themselves and others. Insightful children whose perceptions were rejected by their caregivers learned to consider their own mental processes as thoroughly unacceptable, which allowed them to reconcile their caregiver's behaviour. Years of constant and subtle interactions with controlling, threatening, or neglectful parents created an unusual ability in people with BPD to access and influence the private emotions of others. As children, people who would go on to develop BPD learned to express their desires in a manner that was imperceptible and unthreatening to the people who took care of them. For many of these children, this talent was the only way to get their needs met in dangerous, chaotic, or unsupportive environments. This is how people with BPD can experience distressing symptoms while simultaneously possessing "surprisingly persuasive interpersonal powers." This paradox is unique to the people with the disorder; typically, abuse leads to diminished perceptivity, empathy, and introspection.

According to *Psychological Mindedness*, the talents people with BPD display had been overlooked and underappreciated because they tend to occur in anxious or unsettled individuals who tap into them without conscious effort. If the *DSM* was revised to include mention of these gifts, it would help distinguish BPD from mental illnesses like narcissistic or antisocial personality disorders. Professionals could guard against countertransference, which is when a therapist's psychological needs affect the way they respond to their patients—a pitfall for clinicians who worked with people who could access and strongly influence their private emotions. A strength-based therapeutic approach that validated personal intelligence or giftedness in people with BPD and taught them how to modulate their abnormal sensitivities could impact prognosis, suicide rates, and treatment length for people who were generally viewed poorly.

And perhaps that's why this research is so important. The framing was unprecedented. Scientific articles had never referred to people with BPD as "gifted" before. Instead, the ability to pick up on and take advantage of others' emotions was often described as manipulative. In 2014, researchers from Italy and Chile explored manipulative behaviours in people with BPD to destigmatize their conduct. Manipulation in the clinical realm is often described negatively because it reduces empathy toward the manipulator and undermines the person's search for connection. However, manipulation, influencing others, or—as George calls it—"social engineering" serves people with BPD when it allows them to "achieve a more distinct experience and representation of the other." The 2014 article described a woman with BPD who entered her doctor's consultation room. She watched the doctor "in an interrogative way," sat restlessly, and alternated between remaining silent and answering the therapist's questions in a provocative manner. She explained in a subsequent session that she was testing the doctor's interest in her and his intention and capacity to understand her during bad mental health days.

People with BPD live in a reality that is different from others. Our reality is likely coloured by dysphoria—prolonged, unmotivated, and indistinct feelings that create distressing or uneasy impulses, sensations, and perceptions that invade a person's awareness. In order to overcome dysphoria, the pragmatic move is to manipulate or influence others to better understand other's intentions. People with the disorder are used to being let down by the medical community, framed in highly negative terms, or blamed for the failings of our mental health teams; social engineering allows us to determine if a therapeutic relationship will be safe enough to facilitate healing.

Beyond the windows of Neill's apartment, the snow squalls had slowed to a picturesque fall. Empty beer cans stood sentinel next to the kitchen sink. The conversation had meandered through strategies to handle the emotional crises people with BPD frequently find themselves in, the dynamic between two people with conflicting mental illnesses, and how important it was for the loved ones of people with BPD to tend to their own emotional wellness. My sheet of paper with guiding questions was eventually ignored, left to gather water rings from the bottom of our glasses.

"It's interesting because as perceptive as Miranda can be, there are times when her interpretations are off," M. said. "She'll think a passing glance or change in tone of voice means I'm mad or upset with her when maybe I'm just distracted or out of the present moment."

I knew exactly what M. was referring to. A few days earlier, I asked him a mundane question. His voice dropped into a register I understood as aggravation. I saw frustration fly across his eyes like a comet streaking through the night sky. The corners of his mouth tightened. I burst into tears. Between sobs, I asked him what I had done wrong. He insisted everything was fine. I was determined that it wasn't.

"Our perceptions can definitely be tainted by fear," George said. "We're always worried the other shoe is going to drop."

I nodded. "I'm afraid I'm just one misstep away from being asked to leave. I do everything in my power to prevent that by trying to anticipate your needs. But it takes a lot of energy. Sometimes I make mistakes."

As intuitive as we are, what people with BPD perceive can be distorted by past events. We can experience an incongruity between what we expect to happen and what's actually happening. Researchers have long grappled with this inconsistency, and by the turn of the century, they began to probe emotional recognition biases in people with BPD. Several studies found people with the disorder might be hypersensitive to others' negative emotions in particular. In 1999, psychologist Amy W. Wagner and Marsha M. Linehan determined that women with the disorder were more sensitive to recognizing fear and had trouble accurately appraising neutral facial expressions. A 2004 *Journal of Personality Disorders* study measured preconceptions in social processing by showing participants pictures of emotionally neutral faces and determining how they appraised these faces. People with BPD tended to rate the faces as less friendly and more rejecting. Another study found that people with the disorder had a bias toward perceiving anger but not fear. The participants in this study learned quickly, and their assessments grew more accurate with time. The discrepant results could be reconciled by childhood trauma: people with BPD might be more prone to look for danger due to their early experiences.

In an attempt to clear up these inconsistent findings, clinical psychologist Eric A. Fertuck, whose research focus is BPD, developed a new method for testing how well people with the disorder ascertained the mental states of others. He created the Reading the Mind in the Eyes test (which can be found online should you be interested in your own empathic abilities). Participants were presented with thirty-six black-and-white photos of faces cropped to show only the eye region. They were asked to choose one of four words to describe the mental state of the person in the picture. People with BPD performed better than healthy controls when determining moods associated with both neutral and positive emotions. However, the group with BPD only marginally outperformed healthy controls in reading negative expressions—evidence that negative emotions in others could be misidentified.

In a 2013 evidence review, researchers Natalie Dinsdale and Bernard J. Crespi also tried to explain the inconsistencies in borderline empathy. They hypothesized that one possible cause for the variation in results was the tests used to measure empathy. Some studies used passive stimuli like the Reading the Mind in the Eyes test. Others used interactive stimuli. In addition, a person with BPD's empathetic ability was proposed to differ based on the severity of the disorder or their overall cognitive skills. As Fertuck noted, many studies diverged in how they considered participants' education and intelligence levels, co-occurring mental illnesses, medication status, and where they recruited participants (some were found in hospitals; others in the community). Dinsdale and Crespi found a sufficient amount of evidence for empathetic enhancements in BPD to require further study, but mainly in more interactive experiments. The authors proposed a mix of high levels of attention to social stimuli and dysfunctional social information processing was behind the borderline empathy paradox. People with BPD might be stunted interpersonally because our empathy is in overdrive. We're too sensitive to the moods and feelings of others to properly regulate our interpersonal interactions.

Contradiction is at the core of research about empathy in BPD. But heightened levels of empathy might just be the key to demystifying the poorly understood disorder. Subsequent studies revealed that people with BPD actually felt the emotions of others—as if others' emotions were contagious. This is known as emotional empathy, which can help a person build social connections. Yet people with BPD tend to display poor cognitive empathy, the ability to logically understand others' feelings without reacting, which could align the disorder with other neurodiverse conditions. The BPD empathy paradox could also help differentiate the disorder from other diagnoses like bipolar II. John G. Gunderson, whose early work led to BPD's inclusion in the third edition of the DSM, noted in the second edition of *Borderline Personality Disorder: A Clinical Guide* that people with BPD were more likely to evoke strong empathetic responses from others when compared to people with a bipolar II diagnosis. The answer to the empathy paradox question could shed light on whether or not BPD is actually a personality disorder, or if it is better understood as a developmental or trauma-based disability, which would refine treatment strategies.

The fire had dwindled to pulsing embers. Squirrels scampered along the white streets beyond the window searching for shelter from the icy wind. The spacy looks of exhaustion mixed with the effects of alcohol crept into the faces around the table. But we had become absorbed in our discussion.

I brought up something George had said the last time we spoke—that a relationship between two neurotypical people is like an equal meeting, with each person making up half the relationship. But in a relationship where one person has BPD and the other doesn't, it's more like yin and yang. One partner fit into the other. I asked Neill if he agreed.

"I think that's true. It's the energy George brings to our relationship that can totally motivate me. It's a nice balance. Sometimes I'm the one who gets him going. I love that. We have extremes, but we fire each other up."

M. nodded along, though his eyes were forced shut by a gripping yawn.

"Sometimes people with BPD bring out things in other people that they felt were there," George said, "but didn't know how to express, deal with, or even acknowledge. Everything we feel is in our partner's face. Part of me has learned how to pull out and capitalize on those emotions. We're trying to make everyone feel good and like us. I think it's easy for people with BPD to step up and give large amounts of comfort because we know how shitty it feels to be in a bad place."

The low battery warning on my phone told me it was probably time to wrap the conversation up. The cat snoozed between plush pillows on the couch behind us, his head nestled into his furry paws. M. and I would soon need to brave the frigid wasteland to get back home to our queen-sized bed. I'd recorded two and a half hours of audio—countless hours of transcribing to complete.

I stacked a few glasses and plates filmy with the remnants of food and drink in the crook of my elbow. I headed to the kitchen beyond the chalkboard wall where Neill kept his to-do list and meal plans sketched out. I left the plates next to the sink and grabbed my jacket for a quick vape. In the living room, the guys were still talking about people with BPD and all the wonderful aspects that came from a relationship with an unusual partner.

The screen door creaked shut behind me. The cool night air stung my face and my fingers. Snow swirled beneath the street lights off in the distance. A blast of wind sent my shoulders to my ears. I rocked my knees back and forth—a nervous habit—to shake off the remnants of anxiety I'd begun the night with.

Standing in the cold, I could clearly see the trade-off people with personality disorders or a history of trauma unknowingly engaged in. Despite early studies that indicated abuse can dull empathetic responses, more recent research has explored the intense effects that psychological or physical abuse can have on a person's development and well-being. In 2018, researchers determined that trauma increases attention to emotions and environmental prompts, which can improve the ability to recognize and react to the emotional states of others. The authors confirmed across multiple samples and measures that people who had experienced traumatic events in childhood were more empathetic than adults without trauma histories.

And people with Cluster B personality disorders like BPD, illnesses characterized by dramatic, highly emotional, or unpredictable thinking or behaviour, were more likely to display gifts in certain areas of functioning, despite shortcomings in others. A 2015 study found that elements of some personality disorders were more common in senior business managers at the executive level than in people hospitalized in psychiatric care. The business executives who participated in the study had more characteristics of histrionic and narcissistic personality disorders than the inpatient sample. People with histrionic personality disorder can be charming, dramatic, and expressive—talents that help build relationships. People with narcissistic personality disorder can be highly goal-oriented and ambitious, which can help them climb the corporate ladder. At the same time, these personality disorders can affect a person's social, professional, and romantic relationships.

Ultimately, people who fall under the trauma, personality disorder, or neurodivergent umbrella can be gifted in certain areas but lacking in others. Perhaps, at the end of the day, our abilities balance our deficiencies.

I shivered and took a deep puff of vapour. Maybe it wasn't a matter of deficiency or giftedness. Maybe it was more important to see something positive written about people with the disorder by mental health professionals, who inform how people with BPD are perceived and treated by the general public. BPD is often referred to as one of the hardest illnesses to live with. But hope is the backbone to recovery. People with BPD need to understand that we're not all bad. That we're redeemable. That we're worthy of leading a fulfilling life.

I headed inside to pack up. I had felt tormented by the more problematic aspects of my personality disorder when we'd arrived at Neill's apartment. My inability to socialize because of the pandemic, to expand my perspective, and to see the light in the darkness had left me unmoored. Bundled in my winter gear as I pressed into George and Neill during farewells, I should have felt physically heavy, pulled down by the weight of my clothing. Instead, I felt as light as a balloon on a string. I knew I wasn't going to drift into the tormented sky because I was held firmly by the people I cared about. M. and I trudged into the night hand in hand. I was tired and chilly, but I was smiling. Life with the disorder has its bright spots even during the darkest and coldest evenings.

THE WORLD EXPLODED INTO COLOUR

I hopped out of my grampa Joe's car. My four-year-old legs weren't yet long enough to reach the ground without being airborne for a fraction of a second. My little shoes slapped onto the cracked asphalt of the parking lot in front of a Scarborough strip mall. Bright signs in sharp yellows and screaming reds hovered over a bakery, a moneylender, a rug shop, and a fast-food place all crowded next to each other like too many teeth in a mouth. People milled between shops and hauled bags swollen with purchases back to their vehicles.

Overcome, I sighed and placed a pudgy hand over my chest. I cleared my throat and did the only thing I could think of to release the euphoria bubbling inside my chest. I began to sing the entirety of "A Whole New World" from Disney's 1992 film, *Aladdin*.

Grampa Joe stopped fiddling with his keys. Grandma Kath, or G.K., quit rummaging through her purse. They watched me, this strange child their son had brought home along with his girlfriend. Their faces shifted from perplexed to charmed as I sang. My G.K.'s eyes were watery when I finished the song. Grampa Joe smiled down at me and ruffled my hair. "Come on, Doo Dah. Day's not over yet."

✳

Let's play a game. What would you rather?

1. Emotions that are stable and consistent. You're able to feel pain, sadness, joy, anger—all the stuff that makes us human—but there's a cap on the intensity of these emotions, as if someone's limited the peaks and valleys of an audio wavelength so it won't blow out the speakers.

OR

2. Emotions that exist almost exclusively in extremes with little ability to regulate them. You feel like your loved one is leaving forever when they huff out the door to take a few calming breaths, which summons a pain that radiates across your body in burning ripples. You want to rip your hair out from the roots and claw the flesh from your bones when you're overwhelmed or stressed. But the pendulum swings both ways. You also live with the highest highs and pure moments of unfiltered delight—picture Drew Barrymore laughing in the rain. Sometimes you feel so happy it explodes from your throat in the form of a Disney song.

✳

People with borderline personality disorder feel their emotions deeply. Marsha M. Linehan once likened the emotional sensitivity that people with the disorder experience to having "third-degree burns all over their body." McLean Hospital in Massachusetts, a leader in treating the disorder, notes that "these episodes can also involve extreme feelings of positivity and euphoria."

Perhaps this is why I so often heard my caregivers repeat that Henry Wadsworth Longfellow refrain growing up: "When she was good, / She was very good indeed, / But when she was bad, she was horrid."

Relative to the well-documented detrimental and destructive behaviours of people with BPD, there's a dearth of studies that highlight the positive aspects of the disorder—the spontaneity, the capacity for limitless joy and deep passion, the resiliency, the resourcefulness, the driving urge to find happiness no matter the cost. There are moments when life with BPD is daunting. When it seems that my emotions snap with the strength of an alligator's bite until my solid form is torn into a shuddering mass of snot, tears, blood, and spit. But my joy contains summits as stark as my depths fall.

I walked along worn trails that cut through what had once been thick forest. Sun filtered through the canopy and splashed dabs of light on exposed roots, leafy ferns, and unhurried woolly bear caterpillars. Birds sang cheerful tunes in the summer air.

It was my first or second year at a sleep-away camp in Bracebridge, Ontario. I wouldn't have been older than eleven. My mother's parents had started footing the bill after they sensed that I would benefit from the structure camp provided (unlike my younger brother, who refused the offer and was content to spend his summer holidays poking around at the cottage, chasing our German shepherd, and fishing with his dad).

I climbed the gravel hill that led toward pottery lessons, which were held in a building that was all exposed beams and scarred benches that smelled of acrylic paint and wet clay. Then I felt it. My cheeks were bunched, my lips spread flat, and my mouth pulled tight at the corners. I was smiling. Smiling as hard as I could. Smiling for no reason at all. This was unusual.

A few years earlier, my grade two teacher had sidled up to my desk. She asked me in a low voice why I always seemed so unhappy. Why I never smiled. Was there something going on at home? I scowled to distract the teacher from the blood filling my cheeks and returned to my schoolwork. Yet there I was at camp, plastered with the goofy grin I had seen on so many of my classmates.

I could mostly pretend I was a kid like any other outside the borders of my parents' shadows. (Save for the time a boy I had a crush on asked if I was at camp on "the poor kids' scholarship," or when two counsellors exchanged a withering look of revulsion when I told them my stepdad was a blue-collar worker on disability.) I thrived in the structured days. Meals happened at the same intervals and were followed by singing the same six or seven camp songs. Campers jumped into the lake's chilly waters as soon as we woke up, and we gathered around a fire each evening to close the day. Summer camp was predictable. It was safe. And in that safety was an unfamiliar peace. A peace that made my cheeks bunch, my lips flatten, and pinched the corners of my mouth.

✳

Chasing happiness is what makes us human. Yet the feeling can be elusive, slippery, and hard to hold onto.

It didn't matter what town we were living in, what my cake looked like, or what group of friends I'd managed to cobble together to celebrate my birthday, I always made the same wish. Each year, I inhaled deeply, filled my cheeks with air, closed my eyes, and blew toward the dancing flames. "I wish I was happy," I thought (because you can't tell anyone your wish or it won't come true). And not the fleeting happiness that came when I was with my grandparents or away at summer camp. I wanted happiness that persisted. Happiness that I could bask in. Happiness that wouldn't extinguish so easily as a candle flame.

But people far more fulfilled than me have long struggled with the transient nature of happiness. Abd al-Rahman III was the Caliph of Córdoba during the tenth century; he was a man who knew all flavours of success: military success, political success (he reigned for fifty years), intellectual success, and sexual success (he was said to have kept two separate harems). At the end of his life, he decided to count all the days on which he had felt truly happy. "I have diligently numbered the days of pure and genuine happiness which have fallen to my lot," he wrote. "They amount to Fourteen: —O man! place not thy confidence in this present world!"

✳

Human beings aren't meant to be happy all the time. We've adapted to survive and reproduce as have all creatures on this planet. We probably wouldn't be as effective at enduring if we were content all the time. We wouldn't be motivated to seek what we need or want. We'd be more likely to ignore or overlook threats to our survival. We'd be a bit like Friedrich Nietzsche's "last man" in *Thus Spake Zarathustra*. Described as "the most contemptible thing," the last man was a person who avoided risks at all costs, sought only comfort, and was uninterested in becoming rich or poor because "both are too burdensome." The last man had no taste for negative emotions and instead preferred passive contentment. Zarathustra expected the townspeople to be disgusted when he spoke of the last man. Instead, they called out, "Make us into these last men!"

Difficult emotions like fear or anxiety exist for good reason. They keep us safe from danger and motivate us to engage in adaptive behaviours. Pleasurable emotions prompt us to take action that's likely to increase our well-being or reproductive odds. This push and pull, this back and forth, has allowed our species to last. To achieve. To evolve. Experiencing both ends of the emotional spectrum, regardless of intensity, and adjusting accordingly make us human.

I wasn't an entirely morose child despite what my teacher may have thought. I was happy when I spent the weekend at Granny and Grampa's house. Granny and I sat side by side on the couch, eyes TV-glazed, sipping ginger ale, and munching on Hickory Sticks— my grampa had designed the packaging, which is why Frito-Lay chips filled their cupboards and child-sized plush Hostess Munchies lived in their basement, toys my younger brother liked to practise his wrestling moves on. My grampa would shuffle into the room to tell my granny and me that we looked like two peas in a pod. I was happy when Granny took me to one of my favourite places in the world, McDonald's. She bought me Happy Meals, and we ate salty fries dipped into packets of sticky honey. Or when my bald and bespectacled grampa, who always smelled of Old Spice and cigarette smoke, drove us to the local Chapters. We perused the aisles separately and met at the register. Each of us barely managed to peek over the stacks of books cradled in our arms, which hid our contented grins.

I was happy when Grampa Joe and G.K. took me and my brother away for the weekend; my grandmother got a discount on hotels through her work as a travel agent. Once G.K. smuggled peanuts into African Lion Safari to feed the monkeys. On another trip, our hotel was overbooked and we ended up in a motel in Niagara Falls. Two beautiful ladies in spiked heels shared the room next to ours, but G.K. said we weren't allowed to talk to them, which was too bad since they seemed fun. A lot of men visited their room. On another trip, I played so hard at a waterpark that the soles of my feet looked like raw meat by the end of the afternoon. We frequented a Holiday Inn in Burlington with a bouncy castle so often that my brother and I began to refer to it as "our hotel."

My favourite was when my grandparents or relatives took me to Canada's Wonderland or the Canadian National Exhibition (CNE). I'd ride any terrifying roller coaster the moment I hit the height requirements. I started with the rattly old Ghoster Coaster in Hanna-Barbera Land. I graduated to Thunder Run, a breakneck ride through Wonder Mountain. Next was the Bat's corkscrewed track, Top Gun's simulation of what it feels like to ride an F-14 fighter jet, and the dizzying heights of the drop tower ride at the CNE or the Drop Zone at Wonderland. I gripped the grab bar as tight as I could when I was strapped into my ride of choice and screwed my eyes shut. I was terrified of heights and losing control of my body. I didn't scream as the coaster zoomed toward its end. I froze. My body tensed while it was flung through the air. Most of the time, I was holding my breath without realizing it.

I had learned that my delectable euphoria would surface if I provoked enough fear in myself. I just had to wait for the opposite mood to blow in. I would exit a ride stiff-legged and shaky. The sound of my pounding heart would fade from my ears as the giggles started. Soon, my entire face would be consumed by a smile, and it felt as if someone had released a meadow's worth of butterflies into my chest. I pulled the hand of whoever was with me toward the next ride and skipped along the hot pavement.

This type of thrill-seeking behaviour is common in people with BPD. A 2020 study noted that people with the disorder chase down risky situations (reckless driving, shoplifting, or—if they're a child—roller coasters) because they find them intrinsically rewarding. "Often [people with BPD] seek this kind of excitement to fill their chronic boredom and emptiness, which induces euphoric feelings," the study noted. "It has been speculated that risk-seeking behaviour in BPD may be driven by the desire to stimulate the reward system."

✳

So many of my smiles happened away from home in unfamiliar settings. Perhaps because the act of seeking is key to human fulfillment.

Estonian-American scientist Jaak Panksepp spent his life studying the neuroscience of feelings. In part thanks to his time as a clinical psychology student working in a mental health hospital, Panksepp believed that understanding emotions was the key to developing more effective treatments for psychiatric illnesses. He coined the term *affective neuroscience*, the study of how the brain processes emotions, and he spent much of his professional life mapping out the brain's emotional systems.

In his 1998 book, *Affective Neuroscience: The Foundations of Human and Animal Emotions*, Panksepp documented seven biologically inherited primary emotional command systems: seeking, fear, rage, lust, care, panic or grief, and play. Panksepp argued that seeking was the most important of these core instincts for both humans and animals. When we explore our environments and learn new information that could benefit our survival, our brains reward us with dopamine, the neurotransmitter that allows us to feel pleasure. Panksepp pointed to a lab study in which rats chose to repeatedly electrocute themselves when given access to a lever that caused electric shocks. Panksepp wrote that the rats were motivated by the urge to seek instead of being driven by a reward.

There is early evidence that people with BPD tap into strategies that allow them to prolong joyous experiences. In a 2020 *Journal of Psychopathology and Behavioral Assessment* article, researchers determined that people with the disorder are more likely to savour experiences of joy and use strategies that push away or problem-solve anxiety. This finding indicates that people with BPD might use healthy coping strategies when they experience positive emotions and maladaptive strategies when they feel negative emotions. People with BPD are thought to experience negative emotions more frequently and intensely than positive emotions, which might explain their need to prolong joyous experiences. A 2008 study published in *Acta Psychiatrica Scandinavica* found that people with the disorder got stuck in emotions like sadness, anxiety, and anger. They were less likely to explicitly focus on bringing about positive emotions. This finding aligns with other studies in which individuals with BPD report decreased levels of positive emotional expression compared to healthy controls and people with other mental illnesses.

It makes sense that people who spend so much time in darkness like to bask in the light whenever it shines upon them.

✳

"You did it," I whispered to myself. I was waist-deep in the warm sparkling waters of the Mediterranean. My fingers danced along the sea's surface. I squinted back toward the golden shore. It was dotted with brightly coloured umbrellas, children who played with plastic buckets and shovels in the sand, and women tanning whose oiled arms sheltered their eyes. I smiled so wide in the sunshine I thought my mouth would tear at the corners. The beach, the ocean, the swimmers—the entire world exploded into colours so vibrant they stung my eyes. It was like some invisible force dialed up the saturation of reality. I gasped. I dunked my head beneath the lazy waves and screeched bubbles of delight into the salty ocean.

My aunt had pulled me aside by the elbow a few weeks earlier at a raucous family gathering ahead of my first solo vacation in my early twenties. "Make sure when you're in Greece, you just take a moment to appreciate where you are. That you got there all by yourself. No one helped you. You wanted to experience something, and you worked to save up the money for it."

And I *had* worked to get to the shores of Naxos in the Cyclades Islands. I had spent months meticulously poring over colourful travel guides, carefully budgeting ferry trips between the three islands I planned to visit, booking low-price hostels, and mapping the bus route from the Athens airport to its sweaty and bustling port, Piraeus, before I had left on my two-week trip. I was leaving nothing to chance. It had been three years since my last hospitalization and I still had a tendency to become easily flustered by the unexpected.

Which is exactly what had happened the day before. I was meant to let the *pension* I booked know when my ferry would arrive so they could pick me up. I dialed their number into the scratched and graffitied keypad of a pay phone at the port. The line rang and rang. I called again, but no one answered. I whimpered and paced along scorching sidewalks that stank of urine and pigeon droppings. I turned on my data to send the hosts an email. I constantly refreshed my inbox. Sweat ran down my back in a steady stream. No one replied. My first night in a foreign country and I had nowhere to stay.

At a loss of what else to do, I shuffled onto the ferry with the other passengers. We departed as the sun began its descent beneath the horizon. It illuminated the white buildings nestled into brown hills that the ship steered past. The sky and the sea turned dusky. Sun glitter flashed in the boat's wake. I sipped a rich coffee and looked out the window. The bright-red sun, aglow in washes of golden and pink, slipped behind two dark land masses in the distance.

I told myself I would be fine. I would get off the ferry and wander the port town until I found lodging regardless of cost. I could find cheaper accommodations in the morning. Worst case, I'd sleep on the beach. July temperatures in Naxos average around 27 degrees Celsius.

I would have known I had nothing to fret about had this not been my first visit to Greece in the high tourist season. The ferry's ramp yawned open at my destination and revealed a town nestled in darkness. Illuminated windows danced in the inky hills like fireflies. A group of people waited on the dock. They waved signs for accommodations and yelled over each other about their amenities. Faced with these options, I smiled and hoisted my pack onto one shoulder. "Who can do twenty euros a night or less?" I shouted into the crowd. A small woman whose wild curls were pushed back with a bright-green bandana elbowed her way through the shouters and took my hand. "I'll do twenty for you, but don't tell the French boys in the next room. I charged them forty each."

Underwater, eyes screwed shut against the salt water, I was beyond appreciating where I was or how I got there. I was so happy, so pleased with myself, it felt as if my heart was going to leap through my chest. Before I'd left Canada, I hadn't been sure if I was healthy enough to make it on my own in unfamiliar surroundings where I didn't speak the language. But I had done it. Every cell in my body felt like it was vibrating. I crested the surface. The water droplets on my skin shimmered like diamonds catching the light. A rapturous booming laugh escaped my lips. I beamed in the gentle waters.

✳

Happier people tend to be healthier. One study found that people who experienced more optimistic emotions had greater resistance to the common cold. A 2005 study that examined chronic pain in women determined that those who were more cheerful were less likely to experience physical pain. Wide-ranging research from the Harvard School of Public Health demonstrated that happiness and hopefulness can reduce the risk of heart disease by half. Happiness has a direct correlation to good physical health.

Unhappiness has antithetical results. People with depression have an increased risk of cardiovascular disease, diabetes, stroke, pain, and Alzheimer's disease. Those with BPD are also at risk for chronic diseases, arthritis, and other serious health problems linked to obesity. Traumatic stress in early life can impair brain development and immune systems, and stress response systems.

Of course, happiness doesn't exist in a vacuum. Happiness is impacted by determinants of health like financial stability, social support, access to health services, educational opportunities, experiences of racism, and gender. Aligning with Abraham Maslow's hierarchy of needs theory, a person must have physiological needs met like shelter, food, and warmth before they can satisfy higher needs that bring about peak experiences, or a state of consciousness characterized by euphoria. People with mental illness are less likely to have those basic needs met.

But there's more to happiness than meeting physiological needs. In the Harvard Study of Adult Development, a seventy-five-year study conducted on human happiness, researchers learned that quality interpersonal relationships keep us happier and healthier (also in keeping with Maslow's hierarchy). The people who were most satisfied in their relationships at fifty years old were the healthiest at age eighty. Good relationships act as a protective factor for physical and emotional health.

People who are more isolated are less happy, live shorter lives, and are generally less healthy. Loneliness can kill. Unfortunately, this is an area where people with BPD often struggle. Chaotic and unfulfilling interpersonal relationships are a characteristic that defines the disorder.

Additionally, not everyone with BPD is comfortable basking in their rare sunny moods. I frequent a subreddit about the disorder, and I often come across posts about how happiness can provoke fear or unease. Happiness is regarded as fragile. There's a pervasive feeling that misery is just around the bend. Anxiety that the happiness will soon end or will be replaced by negative events or moods dulls the shine.

This aversion to happiness is known as cherophobia. The feeling can surface as a protective strategy in people with a history of trauma. For example, a child who was punished for being too joyous is more likely to feel uncomfortable when they express positive emotions. Cherophobia is correlated with depression and poor well-being.

People with BPD have poor long-term health odds. Happiness in people with the disorder could be fostered by strengthening social, physical, and emotional supports. People with BPD could add years to their life if they're encouraged to embrace happiness.

*

Ida Storm, a young Norwegian woman diagnosed with BPD (or emotionally unstable personality disorder as the illness is known in Norway), looks straight at the camera she's holding and announces it is April 9, 2011. Behind her, thin trees stretch skyward from the ground scattered with dead leaves. Ida informs her viewers that this day is important because it's the first time in her life that she has bought potatoes.

For eight years, Storm kept a video diary cataloguing her highs and lows to better understand the disorder she lives with, which was made into an award-winning documentary, *Ida's Diary*.

The camera quick-cuts to water boiling in a pot on the stove and then to Ida standing on her porch. She wears a big smile. She jumps up and down in her apartment, washed in soft light, spinning the camera above her head. She's excited about her potatoes and tea. She cheers at her audience and wishes she had someone to hug to share her joy with. A few potatoes rest at the bottom of a pot just beginning to boil. "I'm so proud," she says of her modest achievement. She lounges in front of her bathroom mirror and imagines how fulfilling it would be to have a family to cook potatoes for. Her face glows.

She rests her head in the crook of her arm. Her smile fades a bit as she speaks, at this point, primarily to herself. "Maybe . . . No, I'm sure I'll have [a family] one day."

This is life with BPD. It's not just pain and torment. It can be incomparable joy, triumph over adversity, and finding immense beauty in the overlooked.

✳

The nature of happiness has been debated by philosophers for millennia, but Western culture didn't extol the feeling until the eighteenth century. People didn't necessarily expect happiness as a given before then. It was a novelty. A feeling to be earned through virtue. The shift toward valuing and seeking happiness occurred during the Enlightenment. The reasons for this broad shift are complex. The intellectual and philosophical movement ramped up across Europe, the goals of which were knowledge, freedom, and happiness. Religious notions around suffering and joy evolved. Suffering and sacrifice were no longer the only way to please the Christian god. In his 1689 work, *An Essay Concerning Human Understanding*, John Locke wrote that humans could feel pleasure because God desired the earthly happiness of his creatures.

The Enlightenment was a time of increased comfort for the middle and upper classes. Heating in houses improved, umbrellas were invented, and literacy rates increased. Even dentistry improved, which one historian argues made people more willing to smile. Happiness became more commonplace.

In 1776, the United States Declaration of Independence codified "the pursuit of happiness" as an unalienable right. Some historians believe Thomas Jefferson was inspired to include this right by his favourite philosopher, Locke. In his 1689 essay, Locke uses the phrase "the pursuit of happiness" at least four times. He wrote that "the necessity of pursuing happiness [is] the foundation of liberty."

During the nineteenth century, the goal of happiness made its way into professional and domestic spheres. The idea was that the harder a person worked, the more likely they were to attain higher earnings and social mobility, which was thought to result in more happiness. At home, women were meant to keep the atmosphere light and cheerful to reward their husbands after a long day at work. Parental responsibility also expanded beyond helping children survive to fostering happiness in the home to ensure offspring would grow up to be healthy and normal.

By the 1920s, the happiness industry began to ramp up. Books flooded the market that indicated happiness was a personal responsibility and there were simple steps a person could take to provoke the feeling. The quest for happiness permeated capitalism, inspiring the Happy Meal, television laugh tracks, Disney's happiest place on Earth, the song "Happy Birthday," and much more. Today, the wellness industry market is valued in the trillions. People are still searching for happiness.

In the cloud forests of Panama, a single highway—Route 10—snakes through the village of Hornito in the province of Chiriquí. The hostel I was staying at was built on a sheer hillside and overlooked the dense jungle and quiet mountain town. Most of the structure was partially outdoors except for the bedrooms and basement. The village's pace was slow, but the weather changed in an instant.

I was fresh off another hospitalization. I was out of work. Instead of saving my money, I impulsively travelled to Hornito in the off-season and shared the place with fellow backpackers who had exchanged free lodging for maintenance and custodianship of the hostel—two young men from Argentina and a young woman from Sweden. Occasionally, a person or two would stop in for a night's rest or a break from driving the unending road that cut through the undulating hills. Otherwise, we had the place entirely to ourselves. The hostel had a wraparound wooden deck that offered panoramic views of the valleys below. At that altitude—around 1,100 metres above sea level—the clouds rolled across the sky at astonishing speeds. And so did the weather. Fog, so thick I could hold my hand over the balcony's edge and it would disappear, could clear into a sparkling day in twenty minutes. Storms rolled over the hills behind us, slicked the balcony and mango trees, played a melody on the corrugated roof over the outdoor kitchen, and sent the capuchin monkeys that hung out in a tree in the backyard scampering for shelter. The sky brightened in the time it took to steep a cup of tea to warm my damp bones. Great wet drops splashed to the ground from broad green leaves. Hidden toucans alighted from unseen branches. The neighbouring rooster clucked at a rainbow bending over the horizon.

I spent most of that month in the mountains reading or writing. When I wasn't, I listened to one of the Argentinians croon to his guitar; watched Sanna, the Swedish woman, create a butterfly mosaic from glass fragments on the bathroom wall; played with the momma cat who had given birth to kittens just as I arrived; or wandered down a steep rocky path to visit a local coffee farmer I liked. The hiking was unparalleled. Route 10 was frequented by freight haulers and compact buses that lumbered through the mist. It was often more peaceful to walk the unpaved path.

That's what Sanna and I were doing one sunny afternoon. We had donned our rain jackets (just in case) and wandered beyond the last farm along the dirt road the hostel was on. We followed a trail that led around the neighbour's chicken coop, which the Argentinians had helped build in return for a daily egg delivery. We found ourselves on a cleared patch of land overlooking a tangled jungle.

"There's supposed to be a ravine down this way." Sanna pointed to the greenery below. "We should hear it as we get closer."

We picked along the uncertain terrain, hopped over downed tree trunks, followed dirt switchback trails down deep descents, and stopped to notice a pylon-orange beetle or a bird with a bright-red mohawk. We heard the river and saw flashes of its silver face between tree trunks and thick vines. Sun slivers trickled through the jungle's canopy. Light patterns danced across rocks and roots. We tied our jackets around our waists and chatted about books we liked.

It had all the makings of a glorious and peaceful hike, but part of me was on edge. Jaguars were known to lurk in the jungle. An ex-pat from the next hostel over told me about a girl who was bitten by a vampire bat while she slept and woke in a puddle of her own blood. I had already seen bugs as big as my face. A collection of moths, katydids, and beetles gathered each night beneath the kitchen light like a living painting. I hoped to avoid any poisonous bites. I walked carefully, worried a misstep would send me careening off a ledge. The nearest hospital was an hour away and we had no car.

"We're almost there," Sanna said.

Up ahead, a dark creek shimmered in a break between trees. We bounded down the last few slopes until we'd reached a narrow sandy bank. Sanna took off her shoes and pressed the earth between her toes.

"If we follow the river the way we came, we should find a waterfall," she said. She splashed into the water, which came up to her ankles. I tiptoed in after her. The creek was icy cool on my pale feet.

"It's a bit rocky, isn't it?" I asked. The stream trickled over jagged stones, creating small eddies and rapids. We'd be walking against its flow.

"We can hop from rock to rock."

I looked back toward the overgrown trail we'd followed. I was tempted to turn around but didn't like the thought of traipsing through the jungle alone if Sanna decided to push ahead. Nor did I want to seem cowardly or betray the lack of confidence I had in my body.

Sanna was already traversing the creek. I watched her leap between slippery stones. Her feet found each rock with ease. I followed her footsteps. I wrapped my wet toes around the uneven river rocks and kept my gaze trained on her body's progress.

The stream twisted through the jungle. It gurgled over exposed tree roots and wound its way around leafy ferns and mossy banks. The air was musty and heavy. Up ahead, the water fell over a vertical drop that was chest high.

"Should we turn back?" I asked and nodded toward the impediment.

Sanna shook her white-blonde head. "We can climb up it."

She placed her hands on the rocky ledge. The river split and flowed over her palms. She hoisted herself up and forward. Sanna wriggled like a fish, pulled up a leg, and found her footing. "I'll help you," she said, seeming to sense my nervousness.

She grabbed below my armpits, and I propelled my body upward.

"You got it," she said. I grunted and pulled a leg over. Up ahead, the narrow river continued to gurgle. But beyond it, I heard the roar of water falling from a decent height.

I crept behind Sanna, kept my centre of gravity low, and my hands outstretched. I braced for what I feared was an inevitable fall. We rounded a bend, and the river widened. It gathered into a deep pool fed by a dainty waterfall. Sanna stripped down to her underwear and left her clothes on a mossy log. She waded into the pool, and its dark water crept up to her midriff.

"I'm going under." She dipped her head beneath the fall's torrent. She giggled as she came up and shrieked. "It's cold but so refreshing!"

Our journey upriver and the surprising afternoon humidity had left me clammy. I piled my clothes next to Sanna's and waded through a sandy patch to an underwater slope.

"Just jump in," Sanna said. The water fell around her shoulders like crystal hair. "You'll get used to the temperature faster."

I counted to three in my head and fell awkwardly into the crisp pool. My skin numbed. Sanna beckoned me over. I stood next to her beneath the glacial waterfall yelping and laughing. We lifted our chins and drank straight from the stream. I'd never tasted water so pure. I let the falls pound my shoulders. Nature's massage.

The anxiety my body was riddled with moments earlier had been replaced by joy. We splashed and laughed until our toes were numb, our fingers were wrinkled, and goosebumps swept across our chests.

Buoyed by happiness, the way back down the river was much easier. My step was surer. My pace was more confident. I hopped down the ledge without Sanna's help. We smiled and marvelled over how fortunate we were to find a stream so clear we could kiss our lips to it.

The sky darkened after we headed back up the hill to the hostel. Great grey clouds obscured the sun. A breeze rustled through the trees. Big fat raindrops left dark splotches on the earth. We picked up our pace. Great sheets of rain moved over the hills. We broke into a run, careful to avoid unearthed roots and sharp dips in the gravel road. The rain soaked us.

Back at the hostel, I sat in the kitchen with my hair wrapped in a towel and listened to the rain pound down around us. It occurred to me that my moods were just like the weather at high altitudes. Unpredictable. Extreme. Glorious.

An interesting study landed in my inbox right around the time that I noticed fine lines were appearing on my forehead ahead of my thirty-second birthday. Drawing upon earlier research conducted on people with depression, psychiatrists from Germany discovered that people with BPD who were administered Botox injections had diminished mood swings.

Their findings align with a theory first suggested by Charles Darwin. His facial feedback hypothesis proposed that emotions could be altered by the activity of facial muscles. The German researchers injected Botox into the glabellar region of the face, the lower middle forehead area where negative moods are expressed. This interrupted the communication between the muscles in the forehead and the brain, which changed emotional feedback. Four weeks later, people with BPD in the study had significantly reduced symptoms of the disorder. MRI images showed that Botox had stopped the part of the brain where fears are expressed from activating.

My curiosity was piqued. A quick fix that would curb my negative moods and help me maintain my fading youth? A promise of more positive feelings? An opportunity to choose between stable emotions or unregulated extremes? Sign me up.

But the more I thought about it, the more doubt crept in. Hadn't I already tried to cap the highs and lows of my moods with daily antidepressants? I had rolled the dice on Lexapro at a more daunting time in my life when I'd been willing to forgo the positive if the negative would leave too. I'd been ready to become Nietzsche's last man. But my highs and lows only diminished slightly. What were the odds that I'd get lucky again? Would I be able to keep my unpredictable moments of bliss if I froze the muscles in my forehead?

"The Crab and the Fox" is one of the many fables credited to Aesop, said to be an enslaved storyteller who lived in ancient Greece. A crab chooses to leave the familiar seashore to travel to a lush meadow nearby hoping to feed. Unfortunately, a fox wandering the meadow has the same aim. The fox eats the crab, but before the death bite, the crab laments its choices: "I well deserve my fate, for what business had I on the land, when by my nature and habits I am only adapted for the sea?" The moral of this fable is that contentment with our lot in life is an element of happiness. Between life as an emotional storm or one in which my emotions were largely predictable, I used to always want the latter. Who wouldn't? But I've grown accustomed to moods as jolting as whiplash. Can life with BPD be painful? Absolutely. But it can also be jubilant, ecstatic, and intoxicating. I'll accept the lows if it means I get to keep the highs.

At the end of my life, I won't be able to measure my happiness in days. It's simply impossible for a person who can experience the whole range of human emotions in the span of ten minutes. Instead, I'll count it in hours and minutes. And even if, when all those moments are totalled up, they amount to less than fourteen days, the intensity with which I feel emotions will make it seem like a lot longer.

RECOVERING FROM
AN UNTREATABLE DISORDER

The sun shone over the city's rapidly changing skyline. Its rays fell through a window on the eleventh floor of CAMH's College Street site. I was in the office of the therapist I was referred to after it was suggested that I had borderline personality disorder. The therapist sat cross-legged in her chair. Her brown curls bounced around her shoulders. A clipboard, likely containing notes about me, was balanced on her lap.

"What are your recovery goals, Miranda?" she asked after I explained what had brought me there.

"What do you mean?" I asked.

"What are some of the things you'd like to work on during our time together?"

It was a question that was both simple and daunting. My goal was to feel better. But I couldn't picture what that looked like. The details were blurred. Was recovery fewer panic attacks and thoughts of self-destruction? An ability to return to full-time work? Longer periods between hospitalizations?

I likely answered with some combination of the above, but I remember feeling the answer was insufficient. How could I describe a life without an illness I'd always lived with? It's like asking a person who summoned the courage to hop on a train rolling through town to parts unknown to describe their destination. They might be able to provide broad details like "west" or "the city," but they wouldn't be able to name the local flora and fauna, tell you the best bar in which to drown your sorrows, or reflect with rapture on the smell of freshly cut grass following a harsh winter. Still, I don't fault my therapist for asking about my recovery goals. Because like the choice to hop a train, the contemporary understanding of recovery is that the motivation to heal has to come from within.

Yet, rail travel is an imperfect simile because train routes are primarily linear. There's usually a clear beginning and end of the line. A final destination. A journey from point A to point B. Recovery journeys are rarely that straightforward. It's more common to go from A to C, from C to D, and back to A again. The destination forever shimmers on the horizon.

So, what does recovery from a mental illness actually look like? The American Substance Abuse and Mental Health Services Administration (SAMSHA) offers the most detailed picture. According to the organization, recovery is a "process of change through which individuals improve their health and wellness, live a self-directed life, and strive to reach their full potential." Recovery is supported by secure housing, healthy relationships, and the pursuit of meaningful activities. There are ten principles that help to guide a person's recovery.

1. Hope is the catalyst for the recovery process.
2. Self-determination and self-direction empower individuals to initiate recovery.
3. Paths to recovery are unique and should be highly personalized.
4. Recovery is a holistic process that involves family, self-care practices, housing, employment, transportation, spirituality, primary health care, and more. These services should be accessible and integrated.
5. Recovery is supported by peers and allies who can share experience, knowledge, and skills.
6. Recovery is also supported through larger social networks like family, faith groups, friends, and community members.
7. Honouring culture, values, and traditions are integral to determining a person's recovery journey.
8. Recovery is trauma-informed.
9. Recovery involves taking responsibility. The individual takes responsibility for their personal recovery, families support their loved ones, and communities are responsible for fostering inclusion and addressing discrimination.
10. Recovery is based on respect.

Recovery is a recent option for people with BPD. Historically, people with the disorder were seen as treatment-resistant or unlikely to improve over time.

In a 2008 *Psychiatric Times* article, American psychiatrist Robert J. Gregory said, "It used to be that once borderline personality disorder was diagnosed, the patient was expected never to recover."

BPD diagnoses were linked to treatment resistance since the disorder was first identified by psychoanalyst Adolph Stern in 1938. He noted people with BPD were "extremely difficult to handle effectively by any psychotherapeutic method." In his 1953 Menninger Clinic bulletin, Robert P. Knight determined that people with BPD were unlikely to respond positively to unstructured treatments. The term *negative therapeutic reaction* was used to describe how people with the disorder responded to therapy, which became associated with a generally poor recovery prognosis.

However, timely studies demonstrate that symptom remission occurs in 33 to 99 per cent of people with BPD who receive treatment. Some symptoms associated with the disorder improve even without therapy.

Community-based recovery models date back to at least the seventh century. Europe's oldest recovery-oriented psychiatric community can be found in Geel, Belgium.

The legend begins with Dymphna, the Christian daughter of a pagan king from modern-day County Tyrone, Ireland. Dymphna chose to take a vow of chastity to underscore her devotion to her religion. Her father became mad with grief following her Christian mother's death. His advisers insisted that he marry again, but he would only do so if they could find a bride who was as beautiful and devout as his deceased wife. When no such woman was found, the king turned his eye in the direction of his daughter. Dymphna fled to what is now Geel, where it's said she used her largesse to establish a hospice for people with mental disabilities. But her father used his fortune to track Dymphna down. On May 15, between 620 and 640 CE, he beheaded his fifteen-year-old daughter in the forests of Geel, effectively martyring her.

Dymphna was canonized in 1247. In the mid-fourteenth century, a church was built at her burial site. Rumours spread that people with mental illness who visited it were cured of their symptoms, which were thought to be a punishment from their god. People made pilgrimages to the small village in hopes they would be healed. It became a haven for people with mental illness. And Dymphna was its patron saint. In 1480, a hospice was built close to the church but filled quickly with people seeking relief. Townspeople and local farmers took in pilgrims in need of shelter, some of whom stayed even after their religious observances were completed. A custom was formed and so began a family foster care program that's still in place nearly seven hundred years later.

By 1852, the government took over the program's management from the church. At its height before World War II, nearly four thousand people were in the family foster care system. One in every five residents of Geel had a mental illness. The people who came to Geel for help were referred to as "guests" and not "patients." Guests were paired with a suitable family after a brief period of observation. They were free to participate in the community and contribute to their host household as much as they were able to. Guests became part of a family and of a larger social network. Host families didn't receive much in the way of formal training, but those who were certified to take in boarders saw the designation as a source of pride. Today, the informal community-driven initiative has become an important part of the care the local psychiatric centre provides. The average stay in the foster program is thirty years. Though the number of people staying with foster families has dropped—due to more resources that allow people with mental illness to live independently—the World Health Organization considers Geel "one of the best examples of how communities can become carers of the mentally ill." Geel's secret to success? The community acknowledges each guest's needs will be different and responds by providing meaningful social and work opportunities. More importantly, the families of Geel accept their boarders for who they are and not what they want them to be.

Belonging and acceptance, it seems, are at the heart of recovery.

In the months after my first session with that therapist, my recovery was barely perceptible; my progress, incremental. It was paced no faster than the speed at which I walked to my weekly appointments. I counted the lengths of my breaths while my feet trod from Bloorcourt Village, through Little Italy, just beyond Kensington Market, to the north end of Chinatown to keep myself from dissociating. I counted about fifteen breaths every minute. It took me 675 breaths to walk the distance in one direction. Twice that to come home. And the numbers doubled again when I counted my separate journey to and from group therapy. I counted over ten thousand breaths in the first month of treatment. Countless thousands since.

Mental health recovery involves a lot of numbers for a treatment that's largely unquantifiable. The contemporary philosophy of recovery was popularized by Alcoholics Anonymous, which was founded in the United States in the 1930s. Recovery models were applied to mental health care during the psychiatric survivor/consumer movement of the 1960s and 1970s, which arose from the struggles people with mental illness faced when trying to heal. Mental health recovery takes many forms, some of which rely on measurements not so different from the sobriety coins used in AA. And I've never been very comfortable with numbers. They are too precise. Too exact. Numbers leave no room for error.

Nowhere was this more clearly represented than on the diary card I took home at the end of my DBT skills group meetings. A simple grid was photocopied onto white cardstock. Seven days were counted out with corresponding boxes to track my impulsive urges, how often I acted on the behaviours I wanted to minimize, and if I used any skills to cope with my urges. I kept the card on the freezer door among wedding invitations and flyers for friends' art openings. I dutifully etched a black line onto the card whenever I thought about hurting myself, self-harmed, smoked weed, or felt like smoking it, which was a lot. The card's clean face scarred steadily throughout the week. The numbers rarely plummeted so even when I thought I was having a good day, the card could argue otherwise. The progress I was supposed to be making just wasn't adding up.

Recovery can be frustrating. An approach that helps one person may hinder another. Luckily, the chance to connect with others who had BPD kept me coming back to treatment.

Perhaps one reason people with BPD are still viewed as untreatable, despite evidence to the contrary, is because of the rate at which they drop out of treatment. According to the American Psychological Association, people with BPD quit treatment programs about 70 per cent of the time. Rates of dropout in outpatient DBT can be as high as 24 to 58 per cent. Seven to 54 per cent of people with BPD who try mentalization-based therapy (MBT) don't complete treatment. Schema-focused therapy and transference-focused therapy also have significant dropout rates. More uncomfortable numbers.

Why are dropout rates so high? Mental health professionals have proposed various causes. People with BPD have difficulty maintaining interpersonal relationships and trusting others, which can affect their relationships with therapists. In 2013, researchers determined that people with the disorder who were likely to drop out of DBT treatment had higher levels of anger, more suicide attempts, and poor bonds with their therapists. The method of treatment delivery also impacted dropout rates. A 2021 meta-analysis found that the length of treatment, outpatient settings, and phone coaching all led to higher dropout rates in people with BPD. Reasons for dropout included a lack of motivation, dissatisfaction with treatment, or expulsion.

Therapeutic settings also determined how likely a person with BPD was to stay on the road to recovery. A 2023 study noted that individual therapy tended to have the lowest dropout rates, whereas group therapy had the highest. Therapy for BPD is intensive. Individual therapy can take years. Group therapy takes months and has a rigid schedule. People in my DBT treatment group weren't welcome to return if they missed three sessions. It's a large commitment for even the healthiest of people.

Complicating matters, treatment for BPD is scarce and expensive. A study based in the Netherlands found the yearly cost to treat a person with BPD was approximately twenty-five thousand dollars in 2000, twice as much as it was to treat depression. Studies from the U.K. note that specialized treatment programs like DBT or MBT are routinely underfunded and under-supported. The probability of a DBT treatment team persisting over ten years is under 50 per cent.

But therapy is the best available option for people with BPD. No medication is approved to treat the disorder. There are no quick fixes.

John Thomas Perceval was an early advocate of humane recovery for people with mental illness. He was born to Spencer Perceval, who served as prime minister of the United Kingdom from 1809 until his assassination in 1812. The younger Perceval was just nine years old when he lost his father. The British House of Commons paid fifty thousand pounds to the Perceval family a few days after his father's assassin was hanged. This largesse would later impact Perceval.

As a young man, Perceval entered the army. He saw no combat but developed a preoccupation with religion—early signs of his schizophrenia. By 1830, Perceval had sold his British Army commission and briefly attended the University of Oxford. But whatever purpose he had hoped to find at the institution proved elusive. He left after one term. Perceval travelled to Scotland, where he met with a radical evangelical sect that was said to perform miracles. While he was impressed by their beliefs, members of the group felt Perceval's behaviour was unstable. He travelled to Dublin, where he had sex with a sex worker and became convinced he had contracted syphilis. At this point, Perceval's behaviour was so erratic that he was placed in restraints in the room of the inn where he was staying. His older brother was sent for. In January 1831, Perceval was confined to Brislington and later Ticehurst House, two of England's most expensive private asylums. He spent the next three years in mental institutions.

Perceval memorialized his experience in asylums in two books, which were republished in 1962 as one text, *Perceval's Narrative: A Patient's Account of His Psychosis*. The book catalogued the sadistic treatment he endured. He was chained, manacled, and kept in a straightjacket even while he ate. He was treated primarily with ice baths, a form of hydrotherapy that was thought to combat over-excitement, hypersexuality, and disobedience. Most often, hydrotherapy was used not to heal but to punish. William Handy, a physician at New York Hospital's asylum from 1817 to 1818, recorded fifteen cases in which he used "shower baths" to punish silly behaviour, laughing, tearing clothing, soiling a room, striking staff, or attempting to escape. Perceval's experience with the therapy was no different. He wrote, "I was occasionally seized hand and foot by two men, and thrown suddenly backwards into the bath: and I did not know what need there was for violence, for I never hesitated to enter it. On one occasion, [an attendant] stretched out an iron bar to duck my head under the water by pressing it upon my neck." The beatings administered to Perceval by hospital attendants were equally disturbing, including one that disfigured his ear. At Brislington, he was treated by a surgeon who bled his temporal artery until he nearly fainted. His circumstances improved slightly after he was sent to Ticehurst House, where he spent much of his time petitioning for his release.

Perceval was released in 1834. He married shortly after and began writing about his experiences in 1835. Perceval published his account in 1838. In his opening chapter, he wrote, "I wish to stir up an intelligent and active sympathy, in behalf of the most wretched, the most oppressed, the only helpless of mankind, by proving with how much needless tyranny they are treated and this in mockery by men who pretend indeed their cure, but who are, in reality, their tormentors and destroyers."

Perceval's publishing career was one avenue of mental health treatment reform he pursued. In 1838, he helped to found the Alleged Lunatics' Friend Society. The society sought to protect people with mental illness from unjust confinement and protect those who were confined from cruel and inhumane treatments. It exposed harmful asylums, influenced legislative change, and tried to raise public awareness of how psychiatric practices violated civil liberties. The society campaigned Parliament, the courts, local magistrates, and the public through meetings and lectures. It faced significant difficulties, but its efforts led to gradual changes like more thorough inspections of asylums, clauses in the Lunacy Act of 1845 that safeguarded people in institutions, and the release of many individuals from psychiatric confinement. The society dwindled as its members died off. Today, it's seen as an early iteration of the psychiatric survivors' movement.

And Perceval's efforts have earned him a legacy as a man whose honestness and prescience guided contemporary recovery practices. Look no further than his observations from Ticehurst House: "I deem it is insane conduct on the part of a physician, as any insanity can be in a patient, not to persuade his patients and to prevail upon them to re-enter society suited to their habits, as also not to recommend their friends to place them where such society may be easily procured."

On some days, my recovery looked no different from my illness. One needed only to visit my apartment to gauge this reality. Neon-green pill bottles lined my medicine cabinet. Step-by-step instructions to help me out of a breakdown hung on the fridge.

It was an afternoon like any other. I was writing in the kitchen. Papers were spread across the table. My partner had returned early from his shared office space. But something was off. His tone was clipped. Irritated.

"I know there's something wrong," I said. "How do I fix it?"

He insisted nothing was wrong. He was just stressed from work. But an urgency to maintain the peace eclipsed my ability to hear what my partner said. My focus narrowed to a pinpoint. My emotional instability was a reaction to perceived danger akin to a flight or fight response.

The next few hours would have unfolded very differently had I paused at that moment to assess my feelings. Ideally, I would have asked myself why I felt the need to correct my partner's mood and then practised the DBT skill of opposite action—doing the opposite of what an emotion urged me to do.

Instead, anxiety overtook me. I heaved in my seat. My breath was blocked. My hands and feet tingled with pins and needles. I dug my nails into my palms as hard as I could. I felt nothing. I flapped my arms frantically over the kitchen table. A panic attack. M. froze. His eyes were round with fear.

M. held both palms open like a peace offering. "I'm obviously upsetting you. I'm going to go to the backyard to give you your space, so you can go back to having a nice afternoon."

A small part of me knew this proposed exit was my partner's attempt to calm down. He had to apply his own oxygen mask before he could assist anyone else.

But a primal fear overpowered this insight: my fear of abandonment. I begged him not to go—promised I wouldn't cause any more problems. M. crossed the room to comfort me. But his words were warbled as if he was speaking underwater.

A sweat broke out on the back of my neck. A roar of energy that was smouldering in my gut spread outward. My shoulders locked in their sockets. My arms shook. The adrenaline escaped my body in a guttural scream.

"Let me get you some Ativan," my partner said. He rushed across the apartment to retrieve the medication.

My face was puffy, red, and slicked with tears, drool, and snot. I popped the pill and waited for it to dissipate my panic.

Recovery isn't linear. But I have to keep trying to heal.

Beginning in the 1950s, a new approach to dealing with overcrowded, underfunded, and understaffed mental health asylums swept across North America—deinstitutionalization. Deinstitutionalization was meant to replace long-term psychiatric holds with community-based care for people with mental illness. It was introduced to respond to pressure from the civil rights movement, which included psychiatric survivor advocates. The discovery of psychotropic medications like chlorpromazine (Thorazine) made deinstitutionalization possible, and its cost-effectiveness made it attractive to policy-makers.

Canada's most visible example of deinstitutionalization happened at the Toronto hospital where I'm currently in treatment, located on Queen Street West in the neighbourhood of Parkdale. Back in the 1970s, CAMH was called the Queen Street Mental Health Centre (though it had operated under a variety of names since 1850). The hospital was overcrowded and understaffed, and faced declining standards. According to the *Toronto Star*, "pollution blackened its white brick walls."

In 1979, the nearby provincial Lakeshore Psychiatric Hospital closed its doors and released its patients into the community.

Thousands of people were discharged from the Queen Street centre in the early 1980s under the provincial government's direction. Deinstitutionalization sounded good in theory, but Parkdale had very few community care policies in place for newly discharged people with mental illness. There were few official group homes in the neighbourhood, so former patients ended up in rooming houses or out on the street. In *Landscapes of Despair: From Deinstitutionalization to Homelessness*, authors Michael Dear and Jennifer Wolch write that deinstitutionalization was "a policy adopted with great enthusiasm, even though it was never properly articulated, systematically implemented, nor completely thought through." Parkdale became a poster child of deinstitutionalization gone wrong.

Even today, residents with mental illness (and, by extension, the neighbourhood) face considerable social stigma. As recently as 2000, Parkdale was described by the *Globe and Mail* as "a neighbourhood rife with poverty, drugs, and prostitution . . . broken glass and wild screaming on the street at night. The prostitutes strolling down the sidewalk. The drunks splayed on the grass."

Sometimes community-based mental health care can go very wrong.

Part of what makes BPD recovery complex is the different ways it's conceptualized. Often, recovery from the disorder is defined as symptom remission or no longer meeting its diagnostic criteria. However, people who sought treatment for BPD were found to have hopes beyond symptom reduction. A study of self-generated treatment goals identified improved relationships, a developed sense of self, and better well-being as important aspects of recovery.

Due to these differences, a 2019 qualitative study sought to understand how people with BPD experienced and envisioned recovery. The researchers determined that recovery occurred across three stages. The first stage, described as being stuck, was marked by misdiagnosis, repeated hospitalizations, emotional intensity, and poor self-perception as a result of negative childhood experiences. The second stage began when a person received a BPD diagnosis. Considered a turning point, a diagnosis gave many of the study participants validation and relief, which helped them access the tools they needed to recover. The third and final stage involved improving the experience of people with BPD through developing a greater awareness of emotions and thoughts, strengthening their sense of self, and understanding the perspective of others. Recovery for the participants surveyed didn't necessarily mean a complete reduction in symptoms. Instead, it meant reaching a point where symptoms didn't have such a negative impact on their daily lives.

Four processes were identified that contribute to growth and recovery in people with BPD. The first was an active engagement in the recovery journey. People with BPD had to want and be willing to change in order to begin healing. Hope was seen as crucial to recovery as it assisted with motivation and self-doubt. Engaging in treatment services was another vital factor; however, the people surveyed noted that difficulty accessing fragmented services hindered their recovery. Finally, it was important to people with BPD that they have the opportunity to participate in meaningful activities and relationships, which help foster belonging, self-reflection, and the use of therapeutic skills.

Broad stroke recovery steps are useful to identify, though BPD recovery is as varied as the disorder's presentations. There are multiple paths to healing. A recovery journey is as unique as the individual who is recovering.

The recovery movement in North America has been formalized and refined in the past forty years. Understanding of recovery shifted from clinical definitions (symptom remission, etc.) to holistic approaches that allow a person with mental illness to lead a fulfilling life in the community of their choice.

This approach was brought to the forefront of government policy thanks in large part to advocacy efforts from people with lived experience. In the United States, the Americans with Disabilities Act (ADA) of 1990 gave people with behavioural health disorders the right to live in the community alongside their peers and prohibited discrimination against people with mental illness.

This right was put to the test in the landmark case of Olmstead v. L.C. Two women, Lois Curtis and Elaine Wilson, were voluntarily admitted to the Georgia Regional Hospital's psychiatric unit. Their doctors determined they were ready to move into a community-based program following treatment. However, both women were confined to the institution for several years after their treatment concluded. They filed suit under the ADA to be released. The case went all the way to the Supreme Court. In 1999, the Court determined that the unjustified segregation of persons with disabilities constituted discrimination. People with mental illness had the right to live and receive services in the most integrated setting. This integration mandate helped countless people with behavioural disabilities remain in their homes or communities instead of in institutions.

Throughout the early aughts, agencies like SAMSHA focused on defining what recovery-oriented care looked like and what supports it should include. Models of recovery and care continuums were formalized and piloted in communities. Recovery supports expanded, public education about mental illness gained traction, and access to services improved.

However, a 2021 paper published by Yale University researchers notes, "Over the last ten years, confusion has arisen and limitations have been identified related to notions of recovery . . . threatening further progress toward a recovery orientation and with the potential, perhaps, to turn the clock backward." One such limitation is the perception that recovery is the sole responsibility of the individual. This minimizes the important role mental health services and supports play, the authors argued, and is used as a justification to deny or place limits on these services. For example, people who progress in their recovery may require different supports as their needs evolve, which may not be considered medical necessities. This limits their care. In addition, understanding recovery as a personal journey negates the very real role that determinants of health—like financial stability, safe housing, and freedom from discrimination— play in influencing the course of mental illness.

Canada was a little slower to adopt policies that protected people with mental health disabilities and supported their recovery. Mental health care in the country began to pivot toward recovery-oriented care with the development of the Mental Health Commission of Canada (MHCC) in 2007. The MHCC published a framework for transforming the country's mental health into a recovery-oriented model. The federal government recognized the right of people with mental illness to fully take part in society in 2010 when it ratified the United Nations Convention on the Rights of Persons with Disabilities. This led to the Accessible Canada Act, federal legislation that aims to create a barrier-free country by 2040.

Mental health is recognized as a fundamental aspect of overall well-being, but the Canada Health Act doesn't consider the majority of mental health services offered in the country "medically necessary." This means treatment costs aren't covered under health plans. Recovery can be expensive and, as a result, inaccessible.

When I was growing up, the word *disability* held negative connotations for me. I pictured my stepdad, burnt out and snoring on the couch in front of the television when the word was used. The coffee table messy with an empty chip bag, the cordless phone he spent endless hours on, and an overflowing ashtray. Being a person with a disability in my childhood home meant never working, rarely contributing to the household labour, and having a built-in excuse to be a generally shitty person. It was a state in which a person blamed the world for their problems. And a label that invited others to judge the severity of the disability and question its legitimacy.

It didn't sound like a condition I wanted to experience. Unlike my stepfather's disability, my illness was invisible. There were no pins in my pelvis to point to, no scar stretching across my ass cheek, no limp when bad weather aggravated the pain. Only a troubled mind. A mind that was too tired and daunted to try to prove the depths of its sorrow to a bureaucrat, the type of person I was raised to avoid. No. It was better to deplete my savings or scrape by on part-time work when I was too sick to hold down a full-time job. I had promised myself when I was a child that I would be nothing like my stepdad when I grew up. How could I claim that if I officially shared a label with a man I didn't like or respect?

Therapists and loved ones had suggested I try to register my disability as my illness worsened throughout my adulthood. I always waved them off. The process was too complicated. I was getting by even if I occasionally felt twinges of hunger. I was determined not to be a drain on a system that had never helped me. I believed it never would. I slipped through the cracks too easily and too often.

Ultimately, it wasn't a family member or medical professional who convinced me to claim my disability. It was an accountant.

"Hmm," she said into the phone after I'd walked her through the files that I had emailed to her. "Your yearly income is pretty low."

In the past, I had made excuses to accountants who pointed out my income was well beneath the poverty line. I'd tell them I had a big project coming in and next year would be better. But in 2021, I was too tired to lie. Maybe the pandemic had worn me out. Or maybe all the talk about declining mental health in the news and the community had made it easier to be honest. "I have a mental illness that makes it difficult to work full-time."

I winced and waited for an awkward silence to overtake the line. But the accountant didn't miss a beat. In a slightly bored tone, she recommended applying for the Canada Revenue Agency's disability tax credit. At the very least, it would save me some money, she said.

The accountant's words echoed in my head for six months. I shed some of the shame that I associated with government benefits during that time. The COVID-19 recovery benefit had helped me financially survive the early months of the pandemic when editors weren't sure what the future held and my story assignments dried up. Would applying for a tax credit be so different? The more I considered the matter, the more I became convinced it was a course of action my stepdad would be unlikely to take. He was as irresponsible with his finances as a child with a credit card—more likely to spend money on toys than on necessities. When I called my mother to ask if he received the tax credit, she didn't know. My stepdad's union managed his disability benefits. My parents had never looked into it.

By September 2021, I had filled out the required paperwork, provided copies of my diagnostic reports, and letters of support from my therapist. Within a few months—the wheels of bureaucracy turn slowly—it was done. Letters arrived from the CRA and the National Student Loans Service Centre. My BPD diagnosis constituted a disability in the eyes of the Canadian government. My economic circumstances improved once I accepted my disability. My student loan debt was forgiven. I had a long-term savings plan for the first time in my life. I was able to dedicate more mental space to healing.

Disability, it turned out, wasn't such a bad word. And I had kept my promise to myself. I am nothing like my stepdad.

In their reasoning for publishing *Beyond the Borderline: True Stories of Recovery from Borderline Personality Disorder*, editors John G. Gunderson and Perry D. Hoffman write, "Seldom does an illness, medical or psychiatric, carry such intense stigma and deep shame that its name is whispered, or a euphemism coined, and its sufferers despised and even feared." They refer to BPD as the "leprosy of mental illnesses." The stories contained within the 2016 book are intended to combat myths about the disorder.

Common to so many stories within the book's pages is the agony people with BPD experienced while trying to get their symptoms treated—the stigma, the uncertainty, the misdiagnoses. So much of their recovery journey, and mine, involved educating loved ones and medical professionals about the nature of their diagnosis. And learning how to describe symptoms in a way clinicians and laypeople would recognize. And that's a lot to ask from a person with a debilitating illness.

Perhaps that's just the reality of recovering from BPD. But, maybe, if we tell our stories often enough, if the general public and the people who treat us learn to see us with empathy, and if we underscore our ability to recover, we'll be able to skip all that labour and focus on healing.

*

These days, when I head to CAMH's Queen Street site, I walk through its glass double doors as a guest. Not a patient. I move about the hospital freely. I even have a key card to access locked rooms that would be off-limits to me if I was wearing a gown and a laminated bracelet stamped with my name.

In 2022, I was approved to become a member of Workman Arts, a multidisciplinary arts organization that supports creatives with mental illness. The Workman Arts offices are nestled in CAMH's main building. The organization offers numerous supports to artists and writers, including free office space. It's in the belly of the psychiatric hospital where I wrote significant portions of this book.

The office is sparse. Its only window looks onto a darkened recording studio, which members are welcome to use. The shelves and drawers are empty, devoid of any evidence of the people who use the space when I'm not in it. Very little noise penetrates the beige walls. It's the perfect environment to focus in.

The work happens. The pages fill. I lose track of the effort it takes. I even forget I'm in a hospital. But every so often a Code White sounds over the intercom. I jolt in my seat. Memories of past hospitalizations flood my thoughts. I take a moment and a few deep breaths to reorient myself in the present. Then I return to the work.

ACKNOWLEDGEMENTS

It takes a team of caring and non-judgmental people to help a person with BPD recover. And it takes a caring and non-judgmental team to publish a book about the disorder. Thanks to all the dedicated and tireless people at McClelland & Stewart and Penguin Random House Canada, including Tonia Addison, Crissy Calhoun, Jennifer Griffiths, Sarah Howland, Kimberlee Kemp, Chimedum Ohaegbu, Rebecca Rocillo, and Stephanie Sinclair.

Sincerest thanks to my editor, Haley Cullingham, who championed this collection when it was just a seed of an idea and patiently tended to my words until they grew into something sturdy. Thank you for respecting my disdain for compliments, talking me through the stickier subjects within these pages, and finding the title. You helped turn my dreams into a reality.

Thanks to my agent, the incomparable Samantha Haywood, an excellent advocate and negotiator—I'm grateful you're in my corner. And thanks to Cody Caetano, for his invaluable early feedback on my book proposal.

Early versions of these essays appeared in *Broadview Magazine*, *Xtra*, and my *Life as a Lunatic* newsletter. Thank you to Kristy Woudstra, who helped me find meaning in some of my most painful memories. Thanks to Erica Lenti, the first editor to let me write about living with BPD. Thanks to Caley Moore, who let me explore the world of peer support. And thanks to all the other editors I've worked with over the years who have made me a better writer. Thank you to my subscribers, whose heartfelt feedback keeps me writing on bad days.

Thank you to Yale University's program for recovery and community health and the lived experience leadership fellowship. I'm forever grateful to the Yale faculty, CAMH staff, my mentor, and the co-fellows who supported and encouraged me to write this collection.

Thank you to the writers and researchers who study BPD and whose work and efforts informed so much of this collection. Thank you to people with BPD who have shared their experiences in various forms. This book wouldn't exist without your bravery.

Thanks to the wonderful and patient therapists and counsellors who helped me grow into a version of myself who could pull something like this off: Andrea from Kinark Child and Family Services and Kate from Woodgreen Community Services. My most heartfelt thanks to Emma from CAMH, who has shepherded me from the darkest points of my life to the brightest. I truly would not be where I am without your support, generosity, and guidance.

Thank you to my dear friends, who astound me with their continued love and support: Stacey May Fowles, Scaachi Koul, Rudy Lee, James MacMillan, George August Radosavljevic, Roohi Sahajpal, Alex Sheriff, Michael Stevens, and Amani Waldron. There are surely others whom I've missed—apologies. I'll be a better human now that the book is done. And special thanks to the members of the Breakfast Club, past and present. You all loom so large in my heart.

I'd also like to thank Workman Arts for unfettered use of their office space. And thanks to Wanda (and Dick) O'Hagan for free use of your office and allowing me to adopt you as bonus grandparents. I'm so grateful for your support and friendship.

Thank you to my grandparents, here and gone: Баба and Дідо, Grandma Kay, Granny and Grampa, Grandma Kath and Grampa Joe—you taught me so much and always made me feel so safe and loved. I wouldn't be the person I am without you. Thank you to my kooky aunts, who were always there for the tough conversations. Thank you to my cousins, the twins: I'm so excited to see what the future has in store for you. Thank you to my brother: I'm so proud of you and the life you've made for yourself. And thank you to my mother: you will always be my favourite person.

I can't maintain my reputation as a crazy cat lady without thanking my cats, Pique and Syl, my perfect fluffy supervisors and best little friends. Thank you to Matt, my companion plant. None of this would be possible without your care and support. I love you so much.

Finally, I want to thank people who live with BPD. I see your strengths and your beauty. I hope this book has helped you see them too.

WORKS REFERENCED

PSYCHIC BLEEDING

American Psychiatric Association. *Diagnostic and Statistical Manual of Mental Disorders*. 4th ed., text rev. Washington, D.C.: American Psychiatric Association Publishing, 2000.

American Psychiatric Association. *Diagnostic and Statistical Manual of Mental Disorders*. 3rd ed. Washington, D.C.: American Psychiatric Association Publishing, 1980.

Biskin, Robert S., and Joel Paris. "Comorbidities in Borderline Personality Disorder." *Psychiatric Times* 30, no. 1 (January 2013). https://www.psychiatrictimes.com/view/comorbidities-borderline-personality-disorder.

Bozzatello, Paola, Paola Rocca, Lorenzo Baldassarri, Marco Bosia, and Silvio Bellino. "The Role of Trauma in Early Onset Borderline Personality Disorder: A Biopsychosocial Perspective." *Frontiers in Psychiatry* 12 (September 2021). https://doi.org/10.3389/fpsyt.2021.721361.

Carey, Benedict. "Expert on Mental Illness Reveals Her Own Fight." *The New York Times*, June 23, 2011. https://www.nytimes.com/2011/06/23/health/23lives.html.

Chanen, Andrew M., Henry J. Jackson, Louise K. McCutcheon, Martina Jovev, Paul Dudgeon, Hok Pan Yuen, Dominic Germano et al. "Early Intervention for Adolescents with Borderline Personality Disorder Using Cognitive Analytic Therapy: Randomised Controlled Trial." *British Journal of Psychiatry* 193, no. 6 (December 2008): 477–84. https://doi.org/10.1192/bjp.bp.107.048934.

Dudas, Robert B., Chris Lovejoy, Sarah Cassidy, Carrie Allison, Paula Smith, and Simon Baron-Cohen. "The Overlap between Autistic Spectrum Conditions and Borderline Personality Disorder." *PLOS ONE* 12, no. 9 (September 8, 2017): e0184447. https://doi.org/10.1371/journal.pone.0184447.

Eisendorfer, Arnold. "Adolph Stern 1879–1958." *The Psychoanalytic Quarterly* 28, no. 2 (1959): 149–50. https://doi.org/10.1080/21674086.1959.11926131.

Ervin, Mark, dir. *Futurama.* Season 4, episode 2, "Leela's Homeworld." Aired February 17, 2002, on Fox Network.

Fruzzetti, Alan E. "Why Borderline Personality Disorder Is Misdiagnosed." National Alliance on Mental Illness (blog), October 3, 2007. https://www.nami.org/Blogs/NAMI-Blog/October-2017/Why-Borderline-Personality-Disorder-is-Misdiagnose.

Fyer, Minna R., Allen J. Frances, Timothy Sullivan, Stephen W. Hurt, and John Clarkin. "Comorbidity of Borderline Personality Disorder." *Archives of General Psychiatry* 45, no. 4 (April 1988): 348–52. https://doi.org/10.1001/archpsyc.1988.01800280060008.

Goodman, Marianne, Erin A. Hazlett, Antonia S. New, Harold W. Koenigsberg, and Larry Siever. "Quieting the Affective Storm of Borderline Personality Disorder." *American Journal of Psychiatry* 166, no. 5 (May 2009): 522–28. https://doi.org/10.1176/appi.ajp.2009.08121836.

Gordon, Chris, Mark Lewis, David Knight, and Emma Salter. "Differentiating between Borderline Personality Disorder and Autism Spectrum Disorder." *Mental Health Practice* 23, no. 3 (May 2020): 22–26. https://doi.org/10.7748/mhp.2020.e1456.

Griffiths, Mark. "Validity, Utility and Acceptability of Borderline Personality Disorder Diagnosis in Childhood and Adolescence: Survey of Psychiatrists." *The Psychiatrist* 35, no. 1 (January 2011): 19–22. https://doi.org/10.1192/pb.bp.109.028779.

Guilé, Jean Marc, Laure Boissel, Stéphanie Alaux-Cantin, and Sébastien Garny de La Rivière. "Borderline Personality Disorder in Adolescents: Prevalence, Diagnosis, and Treatment Strategies." *Adolescent Health, Medicine and Therapeutics* 9 (2018): 199–210. https://doi.org/10.2147/AHMT.S156565.

Gunderson, John G., Jonathan E. Kolb, and Virginia Austin. "The Diagnostic Interview for Borderline Patients." *The American Journal of Psychiatry* 138, no. 7 (July 1981): 896–903. https://doi.org/10.1176/ajp.138.7.896.

Gunderson, John G., and Margaret T. Singer. "Defining Borderline Patients: An Overview." *The American Journal of Psychiatry* 132, no. 1 (January 1975): 1–10. https://doi.org/10.1176/ajp.132.1.1.

Hawkins, Ashley A., R. Michael Furr, Elizabeth Mayfield Arnold, Mary Kate Law, Malek Mneimne, and William Fleeson. "The Structure of Borderline Personality Disorder Symptoms: A Multi-Method, Multi-Sample Examination." *Personality Disorders* 5, no. 4 (October 2014): 380–89. https://doi.org/10.1037/per0000086.

Kernberg, Otto. "Borderline Personality Organization." *Journal of the American Psychoanalytic Association* 15, no. 3 (July 1967): 641–85. https://doi.org /10.1177/000306516701500309.

Knight, Robert P. "Borderline States." *Bulletin of the Menninger Clinic* 17, no. 1 (January 1953): 1. https://www.proquest.com/openview/7e8e18cc4db73 fec5da58060fa99a73b.

Linehan, Marsha M. *Building a Life Worth Living: A Memoir.* New York: Random House, 2020.

Linehan, Marsha M., Hubert E. Armstrong, Alejandra Suarez, Douglas Allmon, and Heidi L. Heard. "Cognitive-Behavioral Treatment of Chronically Parasuicidal Borderline Patients." *Archives of General Psychiatry* 48, no. 12 (December 1991): 1060–64. https://doi.org/10.1001/archpsyc.1991.01810360024003.

Membride, Heather. "Mental Health: Early Intervention and Prevention in Children and Young People." *British Journal of Nursing* 25, no. 10 (May 2016): 552–57. https://doi.org/10.12968/bjon.2016.25.10.552.

Park, Lee C., John B. Imboden, Thomas J. Park, Stewart H. Hulse, and H. Thomas Unger. "Giftedness and Psychological Abuse in Borderline Personality Disorder: Their Relevance to Genesis and Treatment." *Journal of Personality Disorders* 6, no. 3 (September 1992): 226–40. https://doi.org/10.1521/pedi.1992.6.3.226.

Porter, C., Jasper Palmier-Claus, Alison Branitsky, Warren Mansell, H. Warwick, and Filippo Varese. "Childhood Adversity and Borderline Personality Disorder: A Meta-Analysis." *Acta Psychiatrica Scandinavica* 141, no. 1 (January 2020): 6–20. https://doi.org/10.1111/acps.13118.

Rosse, Irving C. "Clinical Evidence of Borderland Insanity." *The Journal of Nervous and Mental Disease* 15, no. 10 (October 1890): 669–83. https:// doi.org/10.1097/00005053-189010000-00004.

Ruggero, Camilo J., Mark Zimmerman, Iwona Chelminski, and Diane Young. "Borderline Personality Disorder and the Misdiagnosis of Bipolar Disorder." *Journal of Psychiatric Research* 44, no. 6 (April 2010): 405–8. https://doi.org /10.1016/j.jpsychires.2009.09.011.

Rydén, Göran, Eleonore Rydén, and Jerker Hetta. "Borderline Personality Disorder and Autism Spectrum Disorder in Females: A Cross-Sectional Study." *Clinical Neuropsychiatry* 5, no. 1 (February 2008): 22–30. https://psycnet.apa.org/record/2008-07906-004.

Sansone, Randy A., and Lori A. Sansone. "Gender Patterns in Borderline Personality Disorder." *Innovations in Clinical Neuroscience* 8, no. 5 (May 2011): 16–20. https://www.ncbi.nlm.nih.gov/pmc/articles/PMC3115767.

Sato, Momoko, Peter Fonagy, and Patrick Luyten. "Rejection Sensitivity and Borderline Personality Disorder Features: The Mediating Roles of Attachment Anxiety, Need to Belong, and Self-Criticism." *Journal of Personality Disorders* 34, no. 2 (April 2020): 1–16. https://doi.org/10.1521 /pedi_2019_33_397.

Silverman, David, dir. *The Simpsons*. Season 5, episode 5, "Treehouse of Horror IV." Aired October 28, 1993, on Fox Network.

Stefana, Alberto. *History of Countertransference: From Freud to the British Object Relations School*. Oxfordshire, U.K.: Routledge, 2017.

Stern, Adolph. "Psychoanalytic Investigation of and Therapy in the Border Line Group of Neuroses." *The Psychoanalytic Quarterly* 7, no. 4 (1938): 467–89. https://doi.org/10.1080/21674086.1938.11925367.

Young, Robert, dir. *Jane Eyre*. 1997. London: ITV.

Zanarini, Mary C., Frances R. Frankenburg, Elyse D. Dubo, Amy E. Sickel, Anjana Trikha, Alexandra Levin, and Victoria Reynolds. "Axis I Comorbidity of Borderline Personality Disorder." *American Journal of Psychiatry* 155, no. 12 (December 1998): 1733–39. https://doi.org/10.1176/ajp.155.12.1733.

Zandersen, Maja, and Josef Parnas. "Exploring Schizophrenia Spectrum Psychopathology in Borderline Personality Disorder." *European Archives of Psychiatry and Clinical Neuroscience* 270, no. 8 (July 2020): 969–78. https://doi.org/10.1007/s00406-019-01039-4.

THE BAD GIRLS' SCHOOL

Bowlby, John. *Charles Darwin: A New Biography*. London: Hutchinson, 1991.

Bowlby, John. *A Secure Base: Parent-Child Attachment and Healthy Human Development*. New York: Basic Books, 1988.

Bowlby, John, Mary Ainsworth, Mary Boston, and Dina Rosenbluth. "The Effects of Mother-Child Separation: A Follow-Up Study." *British Journal of Medical Psychology* 29, no. 3–4 (September 1956): 211–47. https://doi.org/10.1111/j.2044-8341.1956.tb00915.x.

Duschinsky, Robbie. "The Emergence of the Disorganized/Disoriented (D) Attachment Classification, 1979–1982." *History of Psychology* 18, no. 1 (February 2015): 32–46. https://doi.org/10.1037/a0038524.

Fonagy, Peter, Tom Leigh, Miriam Steele, Howard Steele, Roger Kennedy, Gretta Mattoon, Mary Target, and Andrew Gerber. "The Relation of Attachment Status, Psychiatric Classification, and Response to Psychotherapy." *Journal of Consulting and Clinical Psychology* 64, no. 1 (February 1996): 22–31. https://doi.org/10.1037/0022-006X.64.1.22.

Gilliam, James E., and David R. Unruh. "The Effects of Baker-Miller Pink on Biological, Physical and Cognitive Behaviour." *Journal of Orthomolecular Medicine* 3, no. 4 (1988): 202–6. https://isom.ca/wp-content/uploads/2020/01/JOM_1988_03_4_11_The_Effects_of_Baker-Miller_Pink_on_Biological_Physical-.pdf.

Gunderson, John G., Mary C. Zarini, Lois W. Choi-Kain, Karen S. Mitchell, Kerry J. Lang, and James I. Hudson. "Family Study of Borderline Personality Disorder and Its Sectors of Psychopathology." *Archives of General Psychiatry* 68, no. 7 (July 2011): 753–62. https://doi.org/10.1001%2Farchgenpsychiatry.2011.65.

Howe, Louise Kapp. *Pink Collar Workers: Inside the World of Women's Work*. New York: G.P. Putnam's Sons, 1977.

Hunt, Gerald. "Sex Differences in a Pink-Collar Occupation." *Industrial Relations* 48, no. 3 (Summer 1993): 441–60. http://www.jstor.org/stable/23073950.

Linehan, Marsha M. *Building a Life Worth Living: A Memoir*. New York: Random House, 2020.

Linehan, Marsha M. *DBT Skills Training Manual*. 2nd ed. New York: Guilford Press, 2014.

Mosquera, Dolores, Anabel Gonzalez, and Andrew M. Leeds. "Early Experience, Structural Dissociation, and Emotional Dysregulation in Borderline Personality Disorder: The Role of Insecure and Disorganized Attachment." *Borderline Personality Disorder and Emotion Dysregulation* 1 (October 2014): 15. https://doi.org/10.1186/2051-6673-1-15.

Porter, C., Jasper Palmier-Claus, Alison Branitsky, Warren Mansell, H. Warwick, and Filippo Varese. "Childhood Adversity and Borderline Personality Disorder: A Meta-Analysis." *Acta Psychiatrica Scandinavica* 141, no. 1 (January 2020): 6–20. https://doi.org/10.1111/acps.13118.

Raphael. *The Madonna of the Pinks ('La Madonna Dei Garofani').* 1506–7. Oil on yew, 27.9 × 22.4 cm. The National Gallery, London. https://www.national gallery.org.uk/paintings/raphael-the-madonna-of-the-pinks-la-madonna -dei-garofani.

Ruocco, Anthony C., Alexander R. Daros, Jie Chang, Achala H. Rodrigo, Jaeger Lam, Justine Ledochowski, and Shelley F. McMain. "Clinical, Personality, and Neurodevelopmental Phenotypes in Borderline Personality Disorder: A Family Study." *Psychological Medicine* 49, no. 12 (September 2019): 2069–80. https://doi.org/10.1017/s0033291718002908.

Schauss, Alexander. "The Physiological Effect of Color on the Suppression of Human Aggression: Research on Baker-Miller Pink." *International Journal of Biosocial Research* 7, no 2. (January 1985): 55–64. https://www.researchgate .net/publication/236843504_The_Physiological_Effect_of_Color_on_the _Suppression_of_Human_Aggression_Research_on_Baker-Miller_Pink.

Wrege, Johannes S., Anthony C. Ruocco, Dean Carcone, Undine E. Lang, Andy C.H. Lee, and Marc Walter. "Facial Emotion Perception in Borderline Personality Disorder: Differential Neural Activation to Ambiguous and Threatening Expressions and Links to Impairments in Self and Interpersonal Functioning." *Journal of Affective Disorders* 284 (April 2021): 126–35. https://doi.org/10.1016/j.jad.2021.01.042.

Zanarini, Mary C., Amy A. Williams, Ruth E. Lewis, R. Bradford Reich, Soledad C. Vera, Margaret F. Marino, Alexandra Levin, Lynne Yong, and Frances R. Frankenburg. "Reported Pathological Childhood Experiences Associated with the Development of Borderline Personality Disorder." *The American Journal of Psychiatry* 154, no. 8 (August 1997): 1101–6. https://doiorg/10.1176 /ajp.154.8.1101.

PINK PLASTIC PLAYHOUSE

DiPaolo, Michael. *Impact of Multiple Childhood Trauma on Homeless Runaway Adolescents.* Oxfordshire, U.K.: Routledge, 2017.

Grabovac, Igor, Lee Smith, Lin Yang, Pinar Soysal, Nicola Veronese, Ahmet Turan Isik, Suzanna Forwood, and Sarah Jackson. "The Relationship between Chronic Diseases and Number of Sexual Partners: An Exploratory Analysis." *BMJ Sexual & Reproductive Health* 46, no. 2 (April 2020): 100–7. https://doi.org/10.1136/bmjsrh-2019-200352.

Health Care for the Homeless Clinicians' Network. "Patients with Borderline Personality Disorders Challenge HCH Clinicians." *Healing Hands* 7, no. 4 (September 2003): 1–3. https://nhchc.org/wp-content/uploads/2019/08/Sept2003HealingHands.pdf.

Ivanich, Jerreed, Melissa Welch-Lazoritz, and Kirk Dombrowski. "The Relationship between Survival Sex and Borderline Personality Disorder Symptoms in a High Risk Female Population." *International Journal of Environmental Research and Public Health* 14, no. 9 (September 2017): 1031. https://doi.org/10.3390/ijerph14091031.

Kellie, Dax J., Khandis R. Blake, and Robert C. Brooks. "What Drives Female Objectification? An Investigation of Appearance-Based Interpersonal Perceptions and the Objectification of Women." *PLOS ONE* 14, no. 8 (August 23, 2019): e0221388. https://doi.org/10.1371/journal.pone.0221388.

Krems, Jaimie Arona, Ahra Ko, Jordan W. Moon, and Michael E.W. Varnum. "Lay Beliefs about Gender and Sexual Behavior: First Evidence for a Pervasive, Robust (but Seemingly Unfounded) Stereotype." *Psychological Science* 32, no. 6 (June 2021): 871–89. https://doi.org/10.1177/0956797620983829.

Maslow, Abraham H. "A Theory of Human Motivation." *Psychological Review* 50, no. 4 (July 1943): 370–96. https://doi.org/10.1037/h0054346.

O'Boyle, Laurie Marie. "The Experience of Abandonment by Persons Diagnosed with Borderline Personality: An Existential-Phenomenological Study." Ph.D. diss., Duquesne University, 2002. https://www.proquest.com/openview/a6db46f6dafee4ef5f2da6a10c16a4a2.

Penner, Francesca, Kiana Wall, Charles Jardin, Jennifer L. Brown, Jessica M. Sales, and Carla Sharp. "A Study of Risky Sexual Behavior, Beliefs about Sexual Behavior, and Sexual Self-Efficacy in Adolescent Inpatients with and without

Borderline Personality Disorder." *Personality Disorders* 10, no. 6 (November 2019): 524–35. https://doi.org/10.1037/per0000348.

Rüsch, Nicolas, Aurelia Hölzer, Christiane Hermann, Elisabeth Schramm, Gitta A. Jacob, Martin Bohus, Klaus Lieb, and Patrick W. Corrigan. "Self-Stigma in Women with Borderline Personality Disorder and Women with Social Phobia." *The Journal of Nervous and Mental Disease* 194, no. 10 (October 2006): 766–73. https://doi.org/10.1097/01.nmd.0000239898.48701.dc.

Sansone, Randy A., and Lori A. Sansone. "Sexual Behavior in Borderline Personality: A Review." *Innovations in Clinical Neuroscience* 8, no. 2 (February 2011): 14–18. https://www.ncbi.nlm.nih.gov/pmc/articles/PMC3071095.

Shaw, Clare, and Gillian Proctor. "Women at the Margins: A Critique of the Diagnosis of Borderline Personality Disorder." *Feminism & Psychology* 15, no. 4 (November 2005): 483–90. https://doi.org/10.1177/0959-353505057620.

Willis, Malachi, and Rosemery O. Nelson-Gray. "Borderline Personality Disorder Traits and Sexual Compliance: A Fear of Abandonment Manipulation." *Personality and Individual Differences* 117 (October 15, 2017): 216–20. https://doi.org/10.1016/j.paid.2017.06.012.

THE DIFFICULT PATIENT

Adler, Gerard. *Borderline Psychopathology and Its Treatment.* New York: Jason Aronson, 1985.

Aviram, Ron B., Beth S. Brodsky, and Barbara Stanley. "Borderline Personality Disorder, Stigma, and Treatment Implications." *Harvard Review of Psychiatry* 14, no. 5 (September–October 2006): 249–56. https://doi.org/10.1080/10673220600975121.

Cleary, Michelle, Nandi Siegfried, and Garry Walter. "Experience, Knowledge and Attitudes of Mental Health Staff Regarding Clients with a Borderline Personality Disorder." *International Journal of Mental Health Nursing* 11, no. 3 (September 2002): 186–91. https://doi.org/10.1046/j.1440-0979.2002.00246.x.

Gunderson, John G. "Borderline Personality Disorder." In *Treatments of*

Psychiatric Disorders, edited by T. Byram Karasu. Washington, D.C.: American Psychiatric Association, 1989: 2749–59.

Herman, Judith Lewis. *Trauma and Recovery*. New York: Basic Books, 1993.

Klein, Pauline, Alicia Kate Fairweather, Sharon Lawn, Helen Margaret Stallman, and Paul Cammell. "Structural Stigma and Its Impact on Healthcare for Consumers with Borderline Personality Disorder: Protocol for a Scoping Review." *Systematic Reviews* 10 (January 2021): 23. https://doi.org/10.1186/s13643-021-01580-1.

Knaak, Stephanie, Andrew C.H. Szeto, Kathryn Fitch, Geeta Mogdill, and Scott Patten. "Stigma towards Borderline Personality Disorder: Effectiveness and Generalizability of an Anti-stigma Program for Healthcare Providers Using a Pre-post Randomized Design." *Borderline Personality Disorder and Emotion Dysregulation* 2 (May 2015): 9. http://dx.doi.org/10.1186/s40479-015-0030-0.

Koekkoek, Bauke, Berno van Meijel, and Giel Hutschemaekers. "'Difficult Patients' in Mental Health Care: A Review." *Psychiatric Services* 57, no. 6 (June 2006): 795–802. https://doi.org/10.1176/ps.2006.57.6.795.

McGrath, Bridget, and Maura Dowling. "Exploring Registered Psychiatric Nurses' Responses towards Service Users with a Diagnosis of Borderline Personality Disorder." *Nursing Research and Practice* 2012 (April 2012): 601918. https://doi.org/10.1155/2012/601918.

Park, Lee C., John B. Imboden, Thomas J. Park, Stewart H. Hulse, and H. Thomas Unger. "Giftedness and Psychological Abuse in Borderline Personality Disorder: Their Relevance to Genesis and Treatment." *Journal of Personality Disorders* 6, no. 3 (September 1992): 226–40. https://doi.org/10.1521/pedi.1992.6.3.226.

Pilkington, Ed. "SlutWalking Gets Rolling after Cop's Loose Talk about Provocative Clothing." *The Guardian*, May 6, 2011. https://www.theguardian.com/world/2011/may/06/slutwalking-policeman-talk-clothing.

Sansone, Randy A., and Lori A. Sansone. "Responses of Mental Health Clinicians to Patients with Borderline Personality Disorder." *Innovations in Clinical Neuroscience* 10, no. 5–6 (May–June 2013): 39–43. https://www.ncbi.nlm.nih.gov/pmc/articles/PMC3719460.

Treloar, Amanda Jane Commons. "A Qualitative Investigation of the Clinician Experience of Working with Borderline Personality Disorder." *New Zealand*

Journal of Psychology 38, no. 2 (2009): 30–34. https://www.psychology.org
.nz/journal-archive/NZJP-Vol382-2009-4-Commons-Treloar.pdf.

Widiger, Thomas A., and Myrna M. Weissman. "Epidemiology of Borderline
Personality Disorder." *Hospital and Community Psychiatry* 42, no. 10
(October 1991): 1015–21. https://doi.org/10.1176/ps.42.10.1015.

Woollaston, K., and P. Hixenbaugh. "Destructive Whirlwind: Nurses' Perceptions
of Patients Diagnosed with Borderline Personality Disorder." *Journal of
Psychiatric and Mental Health Nursing* 15, no. 9 (November 2008): 703–9.
https://doi.org/10.1111/j.1365-2850.2008.01275.x.

Zimmerman, Mark, Louis Rothschild, and Iwona Chelminski. "The Prevalence of
DSM-IV Personality Disorders in Psychiatric Outpatients." *American Journal
of Psychiatry* 162, no. 10 (October 2005): 1911–18. https://doi.org/10.1176
/appi.ajp.162.10.1911.

FATALLY ATTRACTIVE

ABC News. "*Fatal Attraction* Reunion Interview." Uploaded March 6, 2010.
YouTube video, 10:14. https://www.youtube.com/watch?v=31Y8lxu0_yA.

Autytallly. "First off did someone actually say that or did you perceive it that way."
Reddit, May 9, 2022. https://www.reddit.com/r/TrueOffMyChest/comments
/uf5c4w/bpd_and_amber_heard/i7wdsm7.

Ballasy, Nicholas. "Meet the Fans Who Line Up to Watch Johnny Depp Trial
in Person, Including One Who Spent $30k." *People*, May 11, 2022. https://
people.com/movies/fans-witnessing-johnny-depp-amber-heard-trial-in
-person-exclusive.

Baugstø Hanssen, August, dir. *Ida's Diary*. 2014. Oslo: Indie Film. https://vimeo
.com/ondemand/idasdiary.

Benesch, Connie, and Deborah Caulfield. "What's the Attraction Here?: Most-
Talked-About Film of Year Stirs Strong Emotions about Basic Human
Values." *Los Angeles Times*, October 15, 1987. https://www.latimes.com
/archives/la-xpm-1987-10-15-ca-14383-story.html.

Chase, David, creator. *The Sopranos*. 1999–2007. New York: HBO.

Desmarais, Sarah L., Richard A. Van Dorn, Kiersten L. Johnson, Kevin J. Grimm,
Kevin S. Douglas, and Marvin S. Swartz. "Community Violence Perpetration

and Victimization among Adults with Mental Illnesses." *American Journal of Public Health* 104, no. 12 (December 2014): 2342–49. https://doi.org /10.2105/ajph.2013.301680.

Dubinski, Kate. "Five Things Nurse Elizabeth Wettlaufer Suggests Might Have Stopped Her Killing." *CBC News*. August 11, 2018. https://www.cbc .ca/news /canada/london/long-term-care-inquiry-elizabeth-wettlaufer-what-could -have-stopped-you-1.4776403.

Ford, Julian D., and Christine A. Courtois. "Complex PTSD and Borderline Personality Disorder." *Borderline Personality Disorder and Emotion Dysregulation* 8 (May 2021): 16. https://doi.org/10.1186/s40479-021-00155-9.

Fruzzetti, Alan E. "The Impact of Suicide Attempts and Self-Harm on Family Members." Presentation at the 17th Annual Yale NEA BPD Conference: BPD and Life Disrupting Behaviors, online. May 6, 2022.

González, Rafael A., Artemis Igoumenou, Constantinos Kallis, and Jeremy W. Coid. "Borderline Personality Disorder and Violence in the UK Population: Categorical and Dimensional Trait Assessment." *BMC Psychiatry* 16 (June 2016): 180. https://doi.org/10.1186/s12888-016-0885-7.

Göttlich, Martin, Anna Lisa Westermair, Frederike Beyer, Marie Luise Bußmann, Ulrich Schweiger, and Ulrike M. Krämer. "Neural Basis of Shame and Guilt Experience in Women with Borderline Personality Disorder." *European Archives of Psychiatry and Clinical Neuroscience* 270, no. 8 (December 2020): 979–92. https://doi.org/10.1007/s00406-020-01132-z.

Heard, Amber. "I Spoke Up against Sexual Violence and Faced Our Culture's Wrath. That Has to Change." *The Washington Post*, June 2, 2022. https:// www.washingtonpost.com/opinions/ive-seen-how-institutions-protect-men -accused-of-abuse-heres-what-we-can-do/2018/12/18/71fd876a-02ed-11e9 -b5df-5d3874f1ac36_story.html.

I_fought_the_seether. "I'm certainly not saying that Johnny Depp has been a complete angel throughout his life and in his intimate relationships." *Reddit*. May 5, 2022. https://www.reddit.com/r/raisedbyborderlines/comments /ujolc5/what_has_your_experience_been_like_watching_amber/i7fxi3h.

John C. Depp, II v. Amber Laura Heard. CL-2019-2911 (2022). Fairfax Circuit Court, Virginia.

Lyne, Adrian, dir. *Fatal Attraction*. 1987. Los Angeles: Paramount Pictures.

Mangold, James, dir. *Girl, Interrupted*. 1999. Culver City, CA: Columbia Pictures.

Mason, Paul T., and Randi Kreger. *Stop Walking on Eggshells: Taking Your Life Back When Someone You Care about Has Borderline Personality Disorder.* Oakland, CA: New Harbinger Publications, 1998.

Myers, Wade C., Erik Gooch, and J. Reid Meloy. "The Role of Psychopathy and Sexuality in a Female Serial Killer." *Journal of Forensic Sciences* 50, no. 3 (May 2005): 652–57. https://pubmed.ncbi.nlm.nih.gov/15932102/.

Piven, Shira, dir. *Welcome to Me.* 2014. Los Angeles: Alchemy.

Salon Staff. "Mo. Teen Described as Thrill Killer by Prosecutors." *Salon*, February 8, 2012. https://www.salon.com/2012/02/08/mo_teen_described_as_thrill_killer_by_prosecutors_2.

Snyder, Scott. "Pseudologia Fantastica in the Borderline Patient." *The American Journal of Psychiatry* 143, no. 10 (October 1986): 1287–89. https://doi.org/10.1176/ajp.143.10.1287.

Zanarini, Mary C., Frances R. Frankenburg, D. Bradford Reich, Margaret F. Marino, Michelle C. Haynes, and John G. Gunderson. "Violence in the Lives of Adult Borderline Patients." *The Journal of Nervous & Mental Disease* 187, no. 2 (February 1999): 65–71. https://doi.org/10.1097/00005053-199902000-00001.

Zanarini, Mary C., Jolie L. Weingeroff, and Frances R. Frankenburg. "Defense Mechanisms Associated with Borderline Personality Disorder." *Journal of Personality Disorders* 23, no. 2 (April 2009): 113–21. https://doi.org/10.1521/pedi.2009.23.2.113.

COMPANION PLANTS

American Psychiatric Association. *Diagnostic and Statistical Manual of Mental Disorders.* 5th ed., text rev. Washington, D.C.: American Psychiatric Association Publishing, 2022.

Bouchard, Sébastien, and Stéphane Sabourin. "Borderline Personality Disorder and Couple Dysfunctions." *Current Psychiatry Reports* 11, no. 1 (February 2009): 55–62. https://doi.org/10.1007/s11920-009-0009-x.

Bouchard, Sébastien, Stéphane Sabourin, Yvan Lussier, and Evens Villeneuve. "Relationship Quality and Stability in Couples When One Partner Suffers from Borderline Personality Disorder." *Journal of Marital and Family Therapy* 35, no. 4 (October 2009): 446–55. https://doi.org/10.1111 /j.1752-0606.2009.00151.x.

Fertuck, Eric A., Stephanie Fischer, and Joseph Beeney. "Social Cognition and Borderline Personality Disorder." *Psychiatric Clinics of North America* 41, no. 4 (December 2018): 613–32. https://doi.org/10.1016/j.psc.2018.07.003.

Kuhlken, Katherine, Christopher Robertson, Jessica Benson, and Rosemery Nelson-Gray. "The Interaction of Borderline Personality Disorder Symptoms and Relationship Satisfaction in Predicting Affect." *Personality Disorders* 5, no. 1 (January 2014): 20–25. https://doi.org/10.1037/per0000013.

Miano, Annemarie, Luna Grosselli, Stefan Roepke, and Isabel Dziobek. "Emotional Dysregulation in Borderline Personality Disorder and Its Influence on Communication Behavior and Feelings in Romantic Relationships." *Behaviour Research and Therapy* 95 (August 2017): 148–57. https://doi.org/10.1016/j.brat.2017.06.002.

Saxena, Jaya. "Diamonds Aren't Special and Neither Is Your Love." *The Atlantic*, January 29, 2021. https://www.theatlantic.com/family/archive/2021/01 /diamonds-arent-special-and-neither-is-your-love/617859.

Smith, John E. "Time, Times, and the 'Right Time'; 'Chronos' and 'Kairos.'" *The Monist* 53, no. 1 (January 1969): 1–13. http://www.jstor.org/stable/27902109.

Statistics Canada. "'I Don't': Historic Decline in New Marriages during the First Year of the Pandemic." Statistics Canada, November 14, 2022. https:// www150.statcan.gc.ca/n1/daily-quotidien/221114/dq221114b-eng.htm.

Zanarini, Mary C., Jolie L. Weingeroff, and Frances R. Frankenburg. "Defense Mechanisms Associated with Borderline Personality Disorder." *Journal of Personality Disorders* 23, no. 2 (April 2009): 113–21. https://doi.org/10.1521 /pedi.2009.23.2.113.

MOTUS TEMPESTAS

American Psychiatric Association. *Diagnostic and Statistical Manual of Mental Disorders*. 5th ed. Washington, D.C.: American Psychiatric Association Publishing, 2013.

Bakalar, Nicholas. "The Trigger That Makes an Octopus Mom Self-Destruct." *The New York Times*, May 14, 2022. https://www.nytimes.com/2022/05/14 /science/female-octopus-death.html.

Barber, Taylor A., Whitney R. Ringwald, Aidan G.C. Wright, and Stephen B. Manuck. "Borderline Personality Disorder Traits Associate with Midlife Cardiometabolic Risk." *Personality Disorders* 11, no. 2 (March 2020): 151–56. https://doi.org/10.1037/per0000373.

Baumeister, Roy F. "Suicide as Escape from Self." *Psychological Review* 97, no. 1 (January 1990): 90–113. https://doi.org/10.1037/0033-295x.97.1.90.

Brüne, Martin. "Borderline Personality Disorder: Why 'Fast and Furious'?" *Evolution, Medicine, and Public Health* 2016, no. 1 (January 2016): 52–66. https://doi.org/10.1093/emph/eow002.

Brüne, Martin, Valerie Ghiassi, and Hedda Ribbert. "Does Borderline Personality Disorder Reflect the Pathological Extreme of an Adaptive Reproductive Strategy? Insights and Hypotheses from Evolutionary Life-History Theory." *Clinical Neuropsychiatry* 7, no. 1 (February–March 2010): 3–9. https://link .gale.com/apps/doc/A228121873/AONE?u=anon-1fe40269.

Callaway, Ewen. "Snakes Mimic Extinct Species to Avoid Predators." *Nature*, June 11, 2014. https://doi.org/10.1038/nature.2014.15397.

Castle, David J. "The Complexities of the Borderline Patient: How Much More Complex When Considering Physical Health?" *Australasian Psychiatry* 27, no. 6 (December 2019): 552–55. https://doi.org/10.1177/1039856219848833.

Cechak, Paulihna S. "Borderline Personality Disorder: A Review and Analysis Through the Lens of Unified Theory." Ph.D. diss., James Madison University, 2021. https://commons.lib.jmu.edu/diss202029/44.

Chapman, Jennifer, Radia T. Jamil, and Carl Fleisher. *Borderline Personality Disorder*. Tampa, FL: StatPearls Publishing, 2022.

Comtois, Katherine Anne, and Adam Carmel. "Borderline Personality Disorder and High Utilization of Inpatient Psychiatric Hospitalization: Concordance between Research and Clinical Diagnosis." *The Journal of Behavioral Health Services & Research* 43, no. 2 (April 2016): 272–80. https://doi.org/10.1007 /s11414-014-9416-9.

Crowe, Marie. "Never Good Enough—Part 1: Shame or Borderline Personality Disorder?" *Journal of Psychiatric and Mental Health Nursing* 11, no. 3 (June 2004): 327–34. https://doi.org/10.1111/j.1365-2850.2004.00732.x.

Dean, Andy C. "Splitting in Normal and Pathological Populations from the Perspective of Predictive Control Theory." *Theory and Psychology* 14, no. 1 (February 2004): 29–55. https://doi.org/10.1177/0959354304040197.

deCatanzaro, Denys. "Human Suicide: a Biological Perspective." *Behavioral and Brain Sciences* 3, no. 2 (June 1980): 265–72. https://doi.org/10.1017/s0140 525x0000474x.

de la Cruz, John, and Eulito Jr. Vivovicente Casas. "Captive Observation and Comparative Morphology of Philippine Tarsier (*Carlito syrichta*) in Brgy. Hugpa, Biliran, Biliran: A Preliminary Study." *Philippine Journal of Natural Sciences* 20, no. 1 (January 2015): 46–54. https://www.researchgate.net /publication/305390545_Captive_observation_and_comparative_morphology _of_Philippine_tarsier_Carlito_syrichta_in_Brgy_Hugpa_Biliran_Biliran_A _preliminary_study.

Drabble, Jennifer, David P. Bowles, and Lynne Ann Barker. "Investigating the Role of Executive Attentional Control to Self-Harm in a Non-clinical Cohort with Borderline Personality Features." *Frontiers in Behavioral Neuroscience* 8 (August 2014): 274. https://doi.org/10.3389/fnbeh.2014.00274.

Felitti, Vincent J., Robert F. Anda, Dale Nordenberg, David F. Williamson, Alison M. Spitz, Valerie Edwards, Mary P. Koss, and James S. Marks. "Relationship of Childhood Abuse and Household Dysfunction to Many of the Leading Causes of Death in Adults: The Adverse Childhood Experiences (ACE) Study." *American Journal of Preventative Medicine* 14, no. 4 (May 1998): 245–58. https://doi.org/10.1016/S0749-3797(98)00017-8.

Freeman, Kurt A., Rose F. Eagle, Louise S. Merkens, Darryn M. Sikora, Kersti Pettit-Kekel, Mina Nguyen-Driver, and Robert D. Steiner. "Challenging Behavior in Smith-Lemli-Opitz Syndrome." *Cognitive and Behavioral Neurology* 26, no. 1 (March 2013): 23–29. https://doi.org/10.1097/wnn.0b013e31828bf6d5.

Goodman, Marianne, Erin A. Hazlett, Antonia S. New, Harold W. Koenigsberg, and Larry Siever. "Quieting the Affective Storm of Borderline Personality Disorder." *American Journal of Psychiatry* 166, no. 5 (May 2009): 522–28. https://doi.org/10.1176/appi.ajp.2009.08121836.

Gorman, James, and Christopher Whitworth. "How This Beetle Evolved to Mimic Ants." *The New York Times*, April 17, 2018. Video, 3:01. https://www.nytimes .com/video/science/100000005813865/how-this-beetle-evolved-to-mimic -ants.html.

Hamilton, W.D. "The Genetical Evolution of Social Behaviour." *Journal of Theoretical Biology* 7, no. 1 (July 1964): 1–16. https://doi.org/10.1016 /0022-5193(64)90038-4.

Hauschild, Sophie, Dorina Winter, Janine Thome, Lisa Liebke, Christian Schmahl, Martin Bohus, and Stefanie Lis. "Behavioural Mimicry and Loneliness in Borderline Personality Disorder." *Comprehensive Psychiatry* 82 (April 2018): 30–36. https://doi.org/10.1016/j.comppsych.2018.01.005.

Ibáñez, Christian M., and Friedemann Keyl. "Cannibalism in Cephalopods." *Reviews in Fish Biology and Fisheries* 20, no. 1 (March 2010): 123–36. https://doi.org/10.1007/s11160-009-9129-y.

Khosravi, Mohsen. "Eating Disorders among Patients with Borderline Personality Disorder: Understanding the Prevalence and Psychopathology." *Journal of Eating Disorders* 8 (August 2020): 38. https://doi.org/10.1186/s40337 -020-00314-3.

Kienast, Thorsten, Jutta Stoffers, Felix Bermpohl, and Klaus Lieb. "Borderline Personality Disorder and Comorbid Addiction: Epidemiology and Treatment." *Deutsches Arzteblatt International* 111, no. 16 (April 18, 2014): 280–86. https://doi.org/10.3238/arztebl.2014.0280.

Klein, Pauline, Alicia Kate Fairweather, Sharon Lawn, Helen Margaret Stallman, and Paul Cammell. "Structural Stigma and Its Impact on Healthcare for Consumers with Borderline Personality Disorder: Protocol for a Scoping Review." *Systematic Reviews* 10 (January 2021): 23. https://doi.org/10.1186 /s13643-021-01580-1.

Leduc-Cummings, Isabelle, Claire J. Starrs, and J. Christopher Perry. "Idealization." In *Encyclopedia of Personality and Individual Differences*, edited by Todd K. Shackelford and Virgil Zeigler-Hill, 2129–32. New York: Springer Publishing, 2020. https://doi.org/10.1007/978-3-319-24612-3_1385.

Lifjeld, Jan T., Jostein Gohli, Tomáš Albrecht, Eduardo Garcia-del-Rey, Lars Erik Johannessen, Oddmund Kleven, Petter Z. Marki, Taiwo C. Omotoriogun, Melissah Rowe, and Arild Johnsen. "Evolution of Female Promiscuity in Passerides Songbirds." *BMC Evolutionary Biology* 19, no. 169 (2019). https://doi.org/10.1186/s12862-019-1493-1.

Linehan, Marsha M. *Building a Life Worth Living: A Memoir*. New York: Random House, 2020.

Marshall, David C., and Kathy B.R. Hill. "Versatile Aggressive Mimicry of Cicadas by an Australian Predatory Katydid." *PLOS ONE* 4, no. 1 (January 14, 2009): e4185. https://doi.org/10.1371/journal.pone.0004185.

Matzke, Burkhard, Sabine C. Herpertz, Christoph Berger, Monika Fleischer, and Gregor Domes. "Facial Reactions during Emotion Recognition in Borderline Personality Disorder: A Facial Electromyography Study." *Psychopathology* 47, no. 2 (March 2014): 101–10. https://doi.org/10.1159/000351122.

Molina, Juan D., Francisco López-Muñoz, Dan J. Stein, María José Martín-Vázquez, Cecilio Alamo, Iván Lerma-Carrillo, Cristina Andrade-Rosa, María V. Sánchez-López, and Mario de la Calle-Real. "Borderline Personality Disorder: A Review and Reformulation from Evolutionary Theory." *Medical Hypotheses* 73, no. 3 (September 2009): 382–86. https://doi.org/10.1016/j.mehy.2009.03.024.

Mulder, Roger, and Peter Tyrer. "Borderline Personality Disorder: A Spurious Condition Unsupported by Science That Should Be Abandoned." *Journal of the Royal Society of Medicine* 116, no. 4 (April 2023): 148–50. https://doi.org/10.1177/01410768231164780.

Otto, Benjamin, Lisa Kokkelink, and Martin Brüne. "Borderline Personality Disorder in a 'Life History Theory' Perspective: Evidence for a Fast 'Pace-of-Life-Syndrome.'" *Frontiers in Psychology* 12 (July 2021): 715153. https://doi.org/10.3389/fpsyg.2021.715153.

Sansone, Randy A., Jacqueline Barnes, Elizabeth Muennich, and Michael W. Wiederman. "Borderline Personality Symptomatology and Sexual Impulsivity." *The International Journal of Psychiatry in Medicine* 38, no. 1 (March 2008): 53–60. https://doi.org/10.2190/pm.38.1.e.

Sansone, Randy A., and Lori A. Sansone. "The Relationship between Borderline Personality and Obesity." *Innovations in Clinical Neuroscience* 10, no. 4 (April 2013): 36–40. https://www.ncbi.nlm.nih.gov/pmc/articles/PMC3659037/.

Shackleton, Kyle, Hasan Al Toufailia, Nicholas J. Balfour, Fabio S. Nascimento, Denise A. Alves, and Francis L.W. Ratnieks. "Appetite for Self-Destruction: Suicidal Biting as a Nest Defense Strategy in Trigona Stingless Bees." *Behavioral Ecology and Sociobiology* 69, no. 2 (February 2015): 273–81. https://doi.org/10.1007/s00265-014-1840-6.

Society for Humanistic Psychology. "Open Letter to the DSM-5," Society for Humanistic Psychology to the DSM-5 Task Force and the American Psychiatric Association. iPetitions, October 2011. https://www.ipetitions.com/petition/dsm5.

Soloff, Paul H., Patrick Pruitt, Mohit Sharma, Jacqueline Radwan, Richard White, and Vaibhav A. Diwadkar. "Structural Brain Abnormalities and Suicidal Behavior in Borderline Personality Disorder." *Journal of Psychiatric Research* 46, no. 4 (April 2012): 516–25. https://doi.org/10.1016/j.jpsychires.2012.01.003.

Soloff, Paul H., Richard White, and Vaibhav A. Diwadkar. "Impulsivity, Aggression and Brain Structure in High and Low Lethality Suicide Attempters with Borderline Personality Disorder." *Psychiatry Research: Neuroimaging* 222, no. 3 (June 2014): 131–39. https://doi.org/10.1016/j.pscychresns.2014.02.006.

Wang, Z. Yan, Melissa R. Pergande, Clifton W. Ragsdale, and Stephanie M. Cologna. "Steroid Hormones of the Octopus Self-Destruct System." *Current Biology* 32, no. 11 (June 6, 2022): 2572–79. https://doi.org/10.1016/j.cub.2022.04.043.

DANCING ON EGGSHELLS

Barr, Karlen R., Michelle L. Townsend, and Brin F.S. Grenyer. "Using Peer Workers with Lived Experience to Support the Treatment of Borderline Personality Disorder: A Qualitative Study of Consumer, Carer and Clinician Perspectives." *Borderline Personality Disorder and Emotion Dysregulation* 7 (September 2020): 20. https://doi.org/10.1186/s40479-020-00135-5.

Bellamy, Chyrell, Timothy Schmutte, and Larry Davidson. "An Update on the Growing Evidence Base for Peer Support." *Mental Health and Social Inclusion* 21, no. 3 (2017): 161–67. https://doi.org/10.1108/mhsi-03-2017-0014.

Boschma, Geertje, and Courtney Devane. "The Art of Peer Support: Work, Health, Consumer Participation, and New Forms of Citizenship in Late Twentieth-Century Mental Health Care in British Columbia." *BC Studies* 202 (Summer 2019): 65–97. https://link.gale.com/apps/doc/A595705468/AONE?u=anon-f91f9a28.

Canadian Mental Health Association. "Summary of Findings: Mental Health Impacts of COVID-19: Wave 2." Canadian Mental Health Association, 2020. https://cmha.ca/wp-content/uploads/2020/12/CMHA-UBC-wave-2-Summary-of-Findings-FINAL-EN.pdf.

Chang, Cindy J., John K. Kellerman, Kara Binder Fehling, Brian A. Feinstein, and Edward A. Selby. "The Roles of Discrimination and Social Support in the Associations between Outness and Mental Health Outcomes among Sexual Minorities." *American Journal of Orthopsychiatry* 91, no. 5 (2021): 607–16. https://doi.org/10.1037/ort0000562.

Cyr, Céline, Heather Mckee, Mary O'Hagan, and Robyn Priest. "Making the Case for Peer Support." Mental Health Commission of Canada, July 2016. www.mentalhealthcommission.ca/wp-content/uploads/drupal/2016-07/MHCC_Making_the_Case_for_Peer_Support_2016_Eng.pdf.

Davidson, Larry, Chyrell Bellamy, Mathew Chinman, Marianne Farkas, Laysha Ostrow, Judith A. Cook, Jessica A. Jonikas et al. "Revisiting the Rationale and Evidence for Peer Support." *Psychiatric Times* 35, no. 6 (June 29, 2018). https://www.psychiatrictimes.com/view/revisiting-rationale-and-evidence-peer-support.

Davidson, Larry, Chyrell Bellamy, Kimberly Guy, and Rebecca Miller. "Peer Support among Persons with Severe Mental Illnesses: A Review of Evidence and Experience." *World Psychiatry* 11, no. 2 (June 2012): 123–28. https://doi.org/10.1016/j.wpsyc.2012.05.009.

Eubanks-Carter, Catherine, and Marvin R. Goldfried. "The Impact of Client Sexual Orientation and Gender on Clinical Judgments and Diagnosis of Borderline Personality Disorder." *Journal of Clinical Psychology* 62, no. 6 (June 2006): 751–70. https://doi.org/10.1002/jclp.20265.

Favaro, Avis. "Woman with Chemical Sensitivities Chose Medically-Assisted Death after Failed Bid to Get Better Housing." *CTV News*, April 13, 2022. https://www.ctvnews.ca/health/woman-with-chemical-sensitivities-chose-medically-assisted-death-after-failed-bid-to-get-better-housing-1.5860579.

Forchuk, Cheryl, Mary-Lou Martin, Y.L. Chan, and Elsabeth Jensen. "Therapeutic Relationships. from Psychiatric Hospital to Community." *Journal of Psychiatric and Mental Health Nursing* 12, no. 5 (October 2005): 556–64. https://doi.org/10.1111/j.1365-2850.2005.00873.x.

Fox, Daniel J. *Borderline Personality Disorder Workbook: An Integrative Program to Understand and Manage Your BPD*. Oakland, CA: New Harbinger Publications, 2019.

Government of Canada. "Medical Assistance in Dying." Government of Canada, last modified June 1, 2023. https://www.canada.ca/en/health-canada /services/medical-assistance-dying.html.

Hawkins, Ashley A., R. Michael Furr, Elizabeth Mayfield Arnold, Mary Kate Law, Malek Mneimne, and William Fleeson. "The Structure of Borderline Personality Disorder Symptoms: A Multi-Method, Multi-Sample Examination." *Personality Disorders* 5, no. 4 (October 2014): 380–89. https://doi.org/10.1037/per0000086.

Hughes, John, dir. *The Breakfast Club*. 1985. Universal City, CA: Universal Pictures.

Linehan, Marsha M. *Building a Life Worth Living: A Memoir*. New York: Random House, 2020.

Mason, Paul T., and Randi Kreger. *Stop Walking on Eggshells: Taking Your Life Back When Someone You Care about Has Borderline Personality Disorder*. Oakland, CA: New Harbinger Publications, 1998.

Millon, Theodore. *Disorders of Personality: DSM-IV and Beyond*. Hoboken, NJ: Wiley, 1995.

Norling, Darcy C., and Soonie Kim. "Borderline Personality Disorder." In *Handbook of Clinical Psychology Competencies*, edited by Jay C. Thomas and Michel Herson, 877–900. New York: Springer, 2010.

Ontario Human Rights Commission. "Policy on Preventing Discrimination Based on Mental Health Disabilities and Addictions: Appendix A: Historical Context." Ontario Human Rights Commission, June 18, 2014. https:// www.ohrc.on.ca/en/policy-preventing-discrimination-based-mental-health -disabilities-and-addictions/appendix-historical-context.

Paris, Joel. "Suicidality in Borderline Personality Disorder." *Medicina* 55, no. 6 (June 2019): 223. https://doi.org/10.3390/medicina55060223.

Quinn, Gerard, Claudia Mahler, and Olivier De Schutter. "Mandates of the Special Rapporteur on the Rights of Persons with Disabilities; the Independent Expert on the Enjoyment of All Human Rights by Older Persons; and the Special Rapporteur on Extreme Poverty and Human Rights." United Nations Human Rights Office of the High Commissioner, CAN 2/2021, February 3, 2021.

https://spcommreports.ohchr.org/TMResultsBase/DownLoadPublic
CommunicationFile?gId=26002.

Reich, D. Bradford, and Mary C. Zanarini. "Sexual Orientation and Relationship
Choice in Borderline Personality Disorder over Ten Years of Prospective
Follow-Up." *Journal of Personality Disorders* 22, no. 6 (December 2008):
564–72. https://doi.org/10.1521/pedi.2008.22.6.564.

Rodriguez-Seijas, Craig, Theresa A. Morgan, and Mark Zimmerman. "Is There
a Bias in the Diagnosis of Borderline Personality Disorder among Lesbian,
Gay, and Bisexual Patients?" *Assessment* 28, no. 3 (April 2021): 724–38.
https://doi.org/10.1177/1073191120961833.

Runions, Kevin Cecil, Janice Wong, Guilia Pace, and Ivan Salmin. "Borderline
Personality Disorder and Peers: A Scoping Review of Friendship,
Victimization and Aggression Studies." *Adolescent Research Review* 6, no. 4
(December 2021): 359–89. https://doi.org/10.1007/s40894-020-00137-y.

Smits, Maaike L., Dine J. Feenstra, Dawn L. Bales, Jasmijn de Vos, Zwaan Lucas,
Roel Verheul, and Patrick Luyten. "Subtypes of Borderline Personality
Disorder Patients: A Cluster-Analytic Approach." *Borderline Personality
Disorder and Emotion Dysregulation* 4 (July 2017): 16. https://doi.org
/10.1186/s40479-017-0066-4.

Substance Abuse and Mental Health Services Administration. "Core
Competencies for Peer Workers." U.S. Department of Health and Human
Services, last modified February 14, 2022. https://www.samhsa.gov
/brss-tacs/recovery-support-tools/peers/core-competencies-peer-workers.

EXQUISITELY SENSITIVE

Acharya, Tanvi, and Mark Agius. "The Importance of Hope against Other
Factors in the Recovery of Mental Illness." *Psychiatria Danubina* 29,
suppl. 3 (September 2017): 619–22. https://www.psychiatria-danubina.com
/UserDocsImages/pdf/dnb_vol29_noSuppl%203/dnb_vol29_noSuppl%203
619.pdf.

Adler, Gerard. *Borderline Psychopathology and Its Treatment* New York:
Jason Aronson, 1985.

Board, Belinda Jane, and Katarina Fritzon. "Disordered Personalities at Work." *Psychology, Crime & Law* 11, no. 1 (2015): 17–32. https://doi.org/10.1080 /10683160310001634304.

Carter, Linnea, and Donald Rinsley. "Vicissitudes of Empathy in a Borderline Adolescent." *International Review of Psychoanalysis* 4 (1977): 317–26. https://pep-web.org/search/document/IRP.004.0317A.

Chapman, Alexander L., and Kim L. Gratz. *The Borderline Personality Disorder Survival Guide: Everything You Need to Know About Living with BPD.* Oakland, CA: New Harbinger Publications, 2007.

Dinsdale, Natalie, and Bernard J. Crespi. "The Borderline Empathy Paradox: Evidence and Conceptual Models for Empathic Enhancements in Borderline Personality Disorder." *Journal of Personality Disorders* 27, no. 2 (April 2013): 172–95. https://pubmed.ncbi.nlm.nih.gov/23514182.

Domes, Gregor, Daniela Czieschnek, Franziska Weidler, Christoph Berger, Kristina Fast, and Sabine C. Herpertz. "Recognition of Facial Affect in Borderline Personality Disorder." *Journal of Personality Disorders* 22, no. 2 (April 2008): 135–47. https://doi.org/10.1521/pedi.2008.22.2.135.

Fertuck, Eric A., A. Jekal, Inkyung Song, B. Wyman, M.C. Morris, Scott T. Wilson, Beth S. Brodsky, and Barbara Stanley. "Enhanced 'Reading the Mind in the Eyes' in Borderline Personality Disorder Compared to Healthy Controls." *Psychological Medicine* 39, no. 12 (December 2009): 1979–88. https://doi.org /10.1017/s003329170900600x.

Frank, Hallie, and Norman Hoffman. "Borderline Empathy: An Empirical Investigation." *Comprehensive Psychiatry* 27, no. 4 (July–August 1986): 387–95. https://doi.org/10.1016/0010-440x(86)90015-5.

Greenberg, David M., Simon Baron-Cohen, Nora Rosenberg, Peter Fonagy, and Peter J. Rentfrow. "Elevated Empathy in Adults Following Childhood Trauma." *PLOS ONE* 13, no. 10 (October 3, 2018): e0203886. https://doi.org /10.1371/journal.pone.0203886.

Gunderson, John G. "Borderline Personality Disorder." In *Treatments of Psychiatric Disorders*, edited by T. Byram Karasu. Washington, D.C.: American Psychiatric Association, 1989: 2749–59.

Gunderson, John G., and Paul S. Links. *Borderline Personality Disorder: A Clinical Guide.* 2nd ed. Washington, D.C.: American Psychiatric Association Publishing, 2008.

Kernberg, Otto F., Michael A. Selzer, Harold W. Koenigsberg, Arthur C. Carr, and Ann H. Applebaum. *Psychodynamic Psychotherapy of Borderline Patients.* New York: Basic Books, 1989.

Krohn, Alan. "Borderline 'Empathy' and Differentiation of Object Representations: A Contribution to the Psychology of Object Relations." *International Journal of Psychoanalytic Psychotherapy* 3, no. 2 (May 1974): 142–65.

Ladisich, W., and W.B. Feil. "Empathy in Psychiatric Patients." *British Journal of Medical Psychology* 61, no. 2 (June 1988): 155–62. https://doi.org/10.1111 /j.2044-8341.1988.tb02774.x.

Masterson, James F. *Psychotherapy of the Borderline Adult: A Developmental Approach.* Oxfordshire, U.K.: Brunner Mazel, 1976.

Meyer, Björn, Paul A. Pilkonis, and Christopher G. Beevers. "What's in a (Neutral) Face? Personality Disorders, Attachment Styles, and the Appraisal of Ambiguous Social Cues." *Journal of Personality Disorders* 18, no. 4 (August 2004): 320–36. https://doi.org/10.1521/pedi.2004.18.4.320.

Park, Lee C., John B. Imboden, Thomas J. Park, Stewart H. Hulse, and H. Thomas Unger. "Giftedness and Psychological Abuse in Borderline Personality Disorder: Their Relevance to Genesis and Treatment." *Journal of Personality Disorders* 6, no. 3 (September 1992): 226–40. https://doi.org/10.1521 /pedi.1992.6.3.226.

Park, Lee C., and Thomas J. Park. "Personal Intelligence." In *Psychological Mindedness: A Contemporary Understanding,* edited by Mary McCallum and William E. Piper, 133–67. Oxfordshire, U.K.: Routledge, 1997.

Salgado, Rui M., Raquel Pedrosa, and António J. Bastos-Leite. "Dysfunction of Empathy and Related Processes in Borderline Personality Disorder: A Systematic Review." *Harvard Review of Psychiatry* 28, no. 4 (July–August 2020): 238–54. https://doi.org/10.1097/hrp.0000000000000260.

Shapiro, Edward R. "The Psychodynamics and Developmental Psychology of the Borderline Patient: A Review of the Literature." *The American Journal of Psychiatry* 135, no. 11 (November 1978): 1305–15. https://doi.org/10.1176 /ajp.135.11.1305.

Stanghellini, Giovanni. "De-stigmatising Manipulation: An Exercise in Second-Order Empathic Understanding." *South African Journal of Psychiatry* 20, no. 1 (April 2014): 11–14. https://doi.org/10.7196/sajp.510.

Stone, Michael H. "The Course of Borderline Disorders." Presentation at
the American Psychiatric Association Annual Meeting, San Diego, CA,
May 17–22, 1997.

Wagner, Amy W., and Marsha M. Linehan. "Facial Expression Recognition Ability
among Women with Borderline Personality Disorder: Implications for
Emotion Regulation?" *Journal of Personality Disorders* 13, no. 4 (December
1999): 329–44. https://doi.org/10.1521/pedi.1999.13.4.329.

Winter, Dorina, Katrin Koplin, and Stefanie Lis. "Can't Stand the Look in the
Mirror? Self-Awareness Avoidance in Borderline Personality Disorder."
Borderline Personality Disorder and Emotion Dysregulation 2 (November
2015): 13. https://doi.org/10.1186/s40479-015-0034-9.

THE WORLD EXPLODED INTO COLOUR

Aesop. *Aesop's Fables*. Translated by George Fyler Townsend. London: George
Routledge and Sons, 1887.

Baugstø Hanssen, August, dir. *Ida's Diary*. 2014. Oslo: Indie Film. https://vimeo
.com/ondemand/idasdiary.

Callaghan, Shaun, Martin Lösch, Anne Pione, and Warren Teichner. "Feeling
Good: The Future of the $1.5 Trillion Wellness Market." *Our Insights* (blog),
McKinsey & Company Consumer Packaged Goods, April 8, 2021. https://
www.mckinsey.com/industries/consumer-packaged-goods/our-insights
/feeling-good-the-future-of-the-1-5-trillion-wellness-market.

Castle, David J. "The Complexities of the Borderline Patient: How Much More
Complex When Considering Physical Health?" *Australasian Psychiatry* 27,
no. 6 (December 2019): 552–55. https://doi.org/10.1177/1039856219848833.

Chu, Carol, Sarah E. Victor, and E. David Klonsky. "Characterizing Positive and
Negative Emotional Experiences in Young Adults with Borderline Personality
Disorder Symptoms." *Journal of Clinical Psychology* 72, no. 9 (September
2016): 956–65. https://doi.org/10.1002/jclp.22299.

Cohen, Sheldon, William J. Doyle, Ronald B. Turner, Cuneyt M. Alper, and David
P. Skoner. "Emotional Style and Susceptibility to the Common Cold."
Psychosomatic Medicine 65, no. 4 (July 2003): 652–57. https://doi.org/10.1097
/01.psy.0000077508.57784.da.

Darwin, Charles. *The Expression of Emotions in Man and Animals*. London: Murray, 1872.

Davis, Kenneth L., and Christian Montag. "Selected Principles of Pankseppian Affective Neuroscience." *Frontiers in Neuroscience* 12 (2019): 1025. https://doi.org/10.3389/fnins.2018.01025.

Euba, Rafael. "Happy Days—Psychiatry in History." *The British Journal of Psychiatry* 214, no. 6 (June 2019): 328. https://doi.org/10.1192/bjp.2019.92.

Felitti, Vincent J., Robert F. Anda, Dale Nordenberg, David F. Williamson, Alison M. Spitz, Valerie Edwards, Mary P. Koss, and James S. Marks. "Relationship of Childhood Abuse and Household Dysfunction to Many of the Leading Causes of Death in Adults: The Adverse Childhood Experiences (ACE) Study." *American Journal of Preventative Medicine* 14, no. 4 (May 1998): 245–58. https://doi.org/10.1016/S0749-3797(98)00017-8.

Gugliotta, Guy. "For Teeth, It Was France by a Smile." *The Washington Post*, November 26, 2000. https://www.washingtonpost.com/archive/politics/2000/11/26/for-teeth-it-was-france-by-a-smile/28477e4d-7bf3-4538-b4bd-5aee8e7605a8.

Hooley, Jill M., and Sarah R. Masland. "Positive Emotion in Borderline Personality Disorder." In *The Oxford Handbook of Positive Emotion and Psychopathology*, edited by June Gruber, 333–49. New York: Oxford University Press, 2019.

Hüpen, Philippa, Lisa Wagels, Carmen Weidler, Joseph W. Kable, Frank Schneider, and Ute Habel. "Altered Psychophysiological Correlates of Risk-Taking in Borderline Personality Disorder." *Psychophysiology* 57, no. 5 (May 2020): e13540. https://doi.org/10.1111/psyp.13540.

Kruger, Tillmann H.C., Jara Schulze, Agnès Bechinie, Insa Neumann, Stefanie Jung, Christian Sperling, Jannis Engel et al. "Neuronal Effects of Glabellar Botulinum Toxin Injections Using a Valenced Inhibition Task in Borderline Personality Disorder." *Scientific Reports* 12 (August 2022): 14197. https://doi.org/10.1038/s41598-022-17509-0.

Kubzansky, Laura D., and Ichiro Kawachi. "Going to the Heart of the Matter: Do Negative Emotions Cause Coronary Heart Disease?" *Journal of Psychosomatic Research* 48, no. 4–5 (April–May 2000): 323–37. https://doi.org/10.1016/S0022-3999(99)00091-4.

Linehan, Marsha M. *Building a Life Worth Living: A Memoir*. New York: Random House, 2020.

Locke, John. *An Essay Concerning Human Understanding*. Indianapolis: Hacket Publishing, 1996.

Longfellow, Henry Wadsworth. "There was a little girl." Available online at Wikisource, https://en.wikisource.org/wiki/There_Was_a_Little_Girl.

Maslow, Abraham H. "A Theory of Human Motivation." *Psychological Review* 50, no. 4 (July 1943): 370–96. https://doi.org/10.1037/h0054346.

McLean Hospital. "Everything You Need to Know about Borderline Personality Disorder." Mass General Brigham McLean, last modified January 9, 2023. https://www.mcleanhospital.org/essential/bpd.

Mineo, Liz. "Good Genes Are Nice, but Joy Is Better." *The Harvard Gazette*, April 11, 2017. https://news.harvard.edu/gazette/story/2017/04/over-nearly -80-years-harvard-study-has-been-showing-how-to-live-a-healthy-and -happy-life/

National Archives. "Declaration of Independence: A Transcription." U.S. National Archives and Records Administration. https://www.archives.gov/founding -docs/declaration-transcript.

National Institute of Mental Health. "Chronic Illness and Mental Health: Recognizing and Treating Depression." U.S. Department of Health and Human Services, 2021. https://www.nimh.nih.gov/sites/default/files/health /publications/chronic-illness-mental-health/recognizing-and-treating -depression.pdf.

Nietzsche, Friedrich Wilhelm. *Thus Spake Zarathustra*. Translated by Thomas Common. Delhi: Grapevine India, 2019.

Panksepp, Jaak. *Affective Neuroscience: The Foundations of Human and Animal Emotions*. Oxford, U.K.: Oxford University Press, 1998.

Powers, Abigail D., and Thomas F. Oltmanns. "Borderline Personality Pathology and Chronic Health Problems in Later Adulthood: The Mediating Role of Obesity." *Personality Disorders* 4, no. 2 (July 2013): 152–59. https:// doi.org/10.1037/a0028709.

Reisch, Thomas, Ulrich W. Ebner-Priemer, Wolfgang Tschacher, Martin Bohus, and Marsha M. Linehan. "Sequences of Emotions in Patients with Borderline Personality Disorder." *Acta Psychiatrica Scandinavica* 118, no. 1 (July 2008): 42–48. https://doi.org/10.1111/j.1600-0447.2008.01222.x.

Sar, Vedat, Tuğba Türk, and Erdinç Öztürk. "Fear of Happiness among College Students: The Role of Gender, Childhood Psychological Trauma, and Dissociation." *Indian Journal of Psychiatry* 61, no. 4 (July–August 2019): 389. https://doi.org/10.4103/psychiatry.indianjpsychiatry_52_17.

Southward, Matthew W., Stephen A. Semcho, Nicole E. Stumpp, Destiney L. MacLean, and Shannon Sauer-Zavala. "A Day in the Life of Borderline Personality Disorder: A Preliminary Analysis of Within-Day Emotion Generation and Regulation." *Journal of Psychopathology and Behavioral Assessment* 42, no. 4 (December 2020): 702–13. https://doi.org/10.1007/s10862-020-09836-1.

Zautra, Alex J., Lisa M. Johnson, and Mary C. Davis. "Positive Affect as a Source of Resilience for Women in Chronic Pain." *Journal of Consulting and Clinical Psychology* 73, no. 2 (April 2005): 212–20. https://doi.org/10.1037/0022-006x.73.2.212.

RECOVERING FROM AN UNTREATABLE DISORDER

Accessible Canada Act, Statutes of Canada 2019, c. 10. https://laws-lois.justice.gc.ca/eng/acts/a-0.6.

Americans with Disabilities Act of 1990. Public Law 101-336. 101st Congress. July 26, 1990. https://www.congress.gov/bill/101st-congress/senate-bill/933/text.

Arntz, Arnoud, Kyra Mensink, Wouter R. Cox, Rogier E.J. Verhoef, Arnold A.P. van Emmerik, Sophie A. Rameckers, Theresa Badenbach, and Raoul P.P.P. Grasman. "Dropout from Psychological Treatment for Borderline Personality Disorder: A Multilevel Survival Meta-analysis." *Psychological Medicine* 53, no. 3 (February 2023): 668–86. https://doi.org/10.1017%2FS0033291722003634.

Bartram, Mary. "Toward a Shared Vision for Mental Health and Addiction Recovery and Well-Being: An Integrated Two-Continuum Model." *Journal of Recovery in Mental Health* 2, no. 2–3 (Winter–Spring 2019): 55–72. https://jps.library.utoronto.ca/index.php/rmh/article/view/32749.

Bateson, Gregory, ed. *Perceval's Narrative: A Patient's Account of His Psychosis 1830–1832.* London: Hogarth Press, 1962.

Biskin, Robert S. "The Lifetime Course of Borderline Personality Disorder." *The Canadian Journal of Psychiatry* 60, no. 7 (July 2015): 303–8. https://doi.org /10.1177%2F070674371506000702.

Bradbeer, Janice. "Once upon a City: Changing Minds about Mental Illness." *Toronto Star*, May 25, 2017. https://www.thestar.com/yourtoronto/once-upon-a-city-archives/2017/05/25/the-battle-to-change-minds-about-mental-illness.html.

Canada Health Act, Revised Statutes of Canada 1985, c. C-6. https://laws-lois .justice.gc.ca/eng/acts/c-6/page-1.html.

Davidson, Larry. "The Recovery Movement: Implications for Mental Health Care and Enabling People to Participate Fully in Life." *Health Affairs* 35, no. 6 (June 2016): 1091–97. https://doi.org/10.1377/hlthaff.2016.0153.

Davidson, Larry, Michael Rowe, Paul DiLeo, Chyrell Bellamy, and Miriam Delphin-Rittmon. "Recovery-Oriented Systems of Care: A Perspective on the Past, Present, and Future." *Alcohol Research* 41, no. 1 (2021): 09. https:// doi.org/10.35946/arcr.v41.1.09.

Dear, Michael J., and Jennifer R. Wolch. *Landscapes of Despair: From Deinstitutionalization to Homelessness.* Princeton, NJ: Princeton University Press, 1987.

Dingfelder, Sadie F. "Treatment for the 'Untreatable.'" *Monitor on Psychology* 35, no. 3 (March 2004): 46. https://www.apa.org/monitor/mar04/treatment.

Everett, Barbara. "Something Is Happening: The Contemporary Consumer and Psychiatric Survivor Movement in Historical Context." *The Journal of Mind and Behavior* 15, no 1–2, (Winter–Spring 1994): 55–70. http://www.jstor.org /stable/43853632.

Giesen-Bloo, Josephine, Richard van Dyck, Philip Spinhoven, Willem van Tilburg, Carmen Dirksen, Thea van Asselt, Ismay Kremers, Marjon Nadort, and Arnoud Arntz. "Outpatient Psychotherapy for Borderline Personality Disorder." *Archives of General Psychiatry* 63, no. 6 (June 2006): 649–58. https://doi.org/10.1001/archpsyc.63.6.649.

Gunderson, John G., and Perry D. Hoffman. *Beyond the Borderline: True Stories of Recovery from Borderline Personality Disorder.* Oakland, CA: New Harbinger Publications, 2016.

Hervey, Nicholas. "Advocacy or Folly: The Alleged Lunatics' Friend Society, 1845–63." *Medical History* 30, no. 3 (July 1986): 245–75. https://doi.org /10.1017/s0025727300045701.

Iliakis, Evan A., Gabrielle S. Ilagan, and Lois W. Choi-Kain. "Dropout Rates from Psychotherapy Trials for Borderline Personality Disorder: A Meta-analysis." *Personality Disorders* 12, no. 3 (May 2021): 193–206. https://doi.org/10.1037 /per0000453.

Iliakis, Evan A., Anne K.I. Sonley, Gabrielle S. Ilagan, and Lois W. Choi-Kain. "Treatment of Borderline Personality Disorder: Is Supply Adequate to Meet Public Health Needs?" *Psychiatric Services* 70, no. 9 (September 2019): 772–81. https://doi.org/10.1176/appi.ps.201900073.

Knight, Robert P. "Borderline States." *Bulletin of the Menninger Clinic* 17, no. 1 (January 1953): 1. https://www.proquest.com/openview/7e8e18cc4db73fe c5da58060fa99a73b.

Landes, Sara J., Samantha A. Chalker, and Katherine Anne Comtois. "Predicting Dropout in Outpatient Dialectical Behavior Therapy with Patients with Borderline Personality Disorder Receiving Psychiatric Disability." *Borderline Personality Disorder and Emotion Dysregulation* 3 (September 2016): 9. https://doi.org/10.1186/s40479-016-0043-3.

Mental Health Commission of Canada. *Toward Recovery & Well-Being: A Framework for Mental Health Strategy in Canada.* Calgary, AB: Mental Health Commission of Canada, November 2009. https:// mentalhealthcommission.ca/wp-content/uploads/drupal/FNIM_Toward_ Recovery_and_Well_Being_Text_ENG_1.pdf.

Ng, Fiona Y.Y., Marianne E. Bourke, and Brin F.S. Grenyer. "Recovery from Borderline Personality Disorder: A Systematic Review of the Perspectives of Consumers, Clinicians, Family and Carers." *PLOS ONE* 11, no. 8 (August 9, 2016): e0160515. https://doi.org/10.1371/journal.pone.0160515.

Ng, Fiona Y.Y., Michelle L. Townsend, Caitlin E. Miller, Mahlie Jewell, and Brin F.S. Grenyer. "The Lived Experience of Recovery in Borderline Personality Disorder: A Qualitative Study." *Borderline Personality Disorder and Emotion Dysregulation* 6 (May 2019): 10. https://doi.org/10.1186/s40479-019-0107-2.

Olmstead v. L.C., 527 U.S. 581 (1999).

Philp, Margaret. "Researchers Fear Segregating Rich from Poor Will Bring the Ghetto to Canada. Karoline Escaped but Emmy Hasn't Been so Lucky." *The Globe and Mail,* August 5, 2000. https://www.theglobeandmail.com /incoming/researchers-fear-segregating-rich-from-poor-will-bring-the-ghetto- to-canada-karoline-escaped-but-emmy-hasnt-been-so-lucky/article1041562.

Sherer, Richard A. "Personality Disorder: 'Untreatable' Myth Is Challenged." *Psychiatric Times* 25, no. 8 (July 2008). https://www.psychiatrictimes.com /view/personality-disorder-untreatable-myth-challenged.

Silk, Kenneth R. "Augmenting Psychotherapy for Borderline Personality Disorder: The STEPPS Program." *American Journal of Psychiatry* 165, no. 4 (April 2008): 413–15. https://doi.org/10.1176/appi.ajp.2008.08010102.

Stern, Adolph. "Psychoanalytic Investigation of and Therapy in the Border Line Group of Neuroses." *The Psychoanalytic Quarterly* 7, no. 4 (1938): 467–89. https://doi.org/10.1080/21674086.1938.11925367.

Substance Abuse and Mental Health Services Administration. "SAMHSA's Working Definition of Recovery." U.S. Department of Health and Human Services, 2012. https://store.samhsa.gov/sites/default/files/d7/priv/pep12 -recdef.pdf.

Torrey, E. Fuller. *Out of the Shadows: Confronting America's Mental Illness Crisis.* Hoboken, NJ: Wiley, 1998.

United Nations Human Rights Office of the High Commissioner, Convention on the Rights of Persons with Disabilities, A/RES/61/106 (December 13, 2006). https://www.ohchr.org/en/hrbodies/crpd/pages/conventionrights personswithdisabilities.aspx.

van Asselt, A.D.I., C.D. Dirksen, A. Arntz, and J.L. Severens. "The Cost of Borderline Personality Disorder: Societal Cost of Illness in BPD-Patients." *European Psychiatry* 22, no. 6 (September 2007): 354–61. https://doi.org /10.1016/j.eurpsy.2007.04.001.

van Bilsen, Henck P.J.G. "Lessons to Be Learned from the Oldest Community Psychiatric Service in the World: Geel in Belgium." *BJPsych Bulletin* 40, no. 4 (August 2016): 207–11. https://doi.org/10.1192/pb.bp.115.051631.

Vogt, Katharina Sophie, and Paul Norman. "Is Mentalization-Based Therapy Effective in Treating the Symptoms of Borderline Personality Disorder? A Systematic Review." *Psychology and Psychotherapy* 92, no. 4 (December 2019): 441–64. https://doi.org/10.1111/papt.12194.

Wnuk, Susan, Shelley McMain, Paul S. Links, Liat Habinski, Joshua Murray, and Tim Guimond. "Factors Related to Dropout from Treatment in Two Outpatient Treatments for Borderline Personality Disorder." *Journal of*